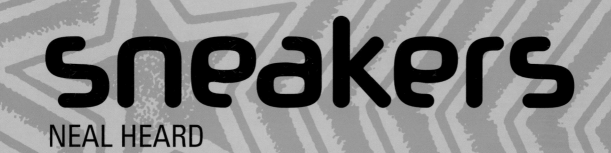

sneakers

NEAL HEARD

THIS IS A CARLTON BOOK

Text and design copyright © 2003
Carlton Books Limited
Special photography © David Gill

This paperback edition published
by Carlton Books Limited 2005
20 Mortimer Street
London W1T 3JW

Executive Editor: Lisa Dyer
Design: Zoë Dissell
Copy Editor: Jonathan Hilton
Photographer: David Gill
Picture Editor: Elena Goodinson
Production: Lucy Woodhead
and Caroline Alberti

ISBN 1 84442 483 9

Printed and bound in China

Many thanks go to Robert Brooks, Jeremy Howlett, Helen Sweeney-
Dougan, Remi Kabaka, Kevin Hurry and Neal Heard for supplying their
footwear. Many thanks also go to Russell Porter for the Back to the
Future photographs.

Love to Ricky and Scarlett, Mam and Dad, J and E, and cheers to Idris
Kaid and Fraser Moss for letting me in and to Matthew Griffo Griffiths
for sharing the adventure and love of the trainers.

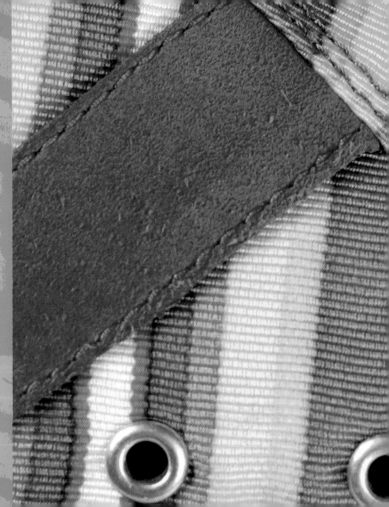

sneakers

NEAL HEARD

CARLTON BOOKS

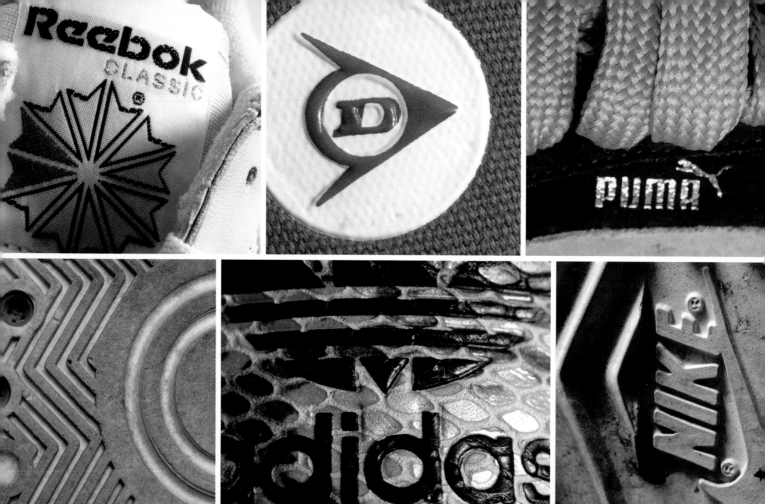

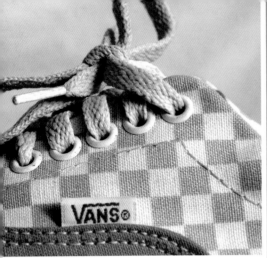

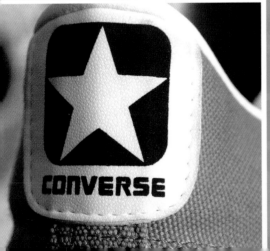

contents

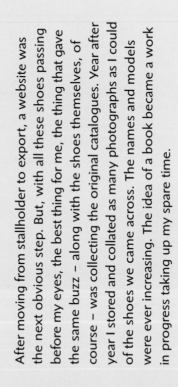

foreword
NEAL HEARD

I love trainers. I always have, and I always will. Growing up as a soccer-mad teenager in the early 1980s, what choice did I have? It was almost a prerequisite to love your footwear.

I have been lucky enough to have spent the best part of the last decade working with and around trainers. What started out as a shared hobby, looking for old deadstock trainers, shoes that were no longer on release, became my full-time occupation.

After moving from stallholder to export, a website was the next obvious step. But, with all these shoes passing before my eyes, the best thing for me, the thing that gave the same buzz – along with the shoes themselves, of course – was collecting the original catalogues. Year after year I stored and collated as many photographs as I could of the shoes we came across. The names and models were ever increasing. The idea of a book became a work in progress taking up my spare time.

A book on trainers... it's something I have wanted to put together for years. Like many other trainer lovers, I fell into the habit of keeping and filing every article on trainers and trainer culture I came across. It was like an obsession, and I could not get enough. However, the explosion in the popularity of the culture still took me by surprise, but what was even more surprising was that, despite the popular appetite for all things 'trainer' – or 'sneaker' if you're North American – there seemed to be very little material written about the shoes themselves. It is only fairly recently that the brands have woken up to their own histories and stories and have seriously started to collate the information they have in their archives.

Whatever happened, I thought the task would be fairly simple. The book should be about the trainers, containing as many photographs as possible of the rare and sought-after models. I also wanted the book to reflect something of the 'ordinary' people who love these shoes for themselves and always will. In the end, the book has taken a great deal of time and effort to produce and there are many people I would like to thank, for without their help it would not have been possible. Particularly I would like to thank Helen Sweeney-Dougan for her considerable input, connections and shoes, and also big thanks to collectors Robert Brooks and Jeremy Howlett. As for all the other collectors who supplied their treasured shoes to be photographed, and the others who offered their expertise on certain chapters, I point you towards the contributors' page for their details.

I can only hope that I have done justice to this fascinating subject and that, whatever your loyalties or brand allegiances, the book speaks to you in some way.

Read on, and enjoy.

introduction

In life, more often than not, the first cut is the deepest. This old saying can certainly be used to describe my feelings for the first pair of trainers that left a mark on me – a pair of Adidas ZX250s.

Stumbling through dark, cramped side streets on a grim, winter's afternoon, heading toward the hallowed turf of my local soccer ground, through the crowds of lads strutting as proud as peacocks I see them. The hit is immediate. Welcome, to the world of Trainer Obsession.

There was something hypnotic about the whole package. The colours, the logo, the contrasting shiny nylon and suede materials – and later on, even the box – struck a cord deep within. These trainers were not just for wearing to run or kick in; they were more than that. They were items of desire, beauty... something I just had to possess. From that day on, trainers had taken a hold on me, and the grip is as strong today as it was way back then.

That was Britain in the early 1980s; it was the era of the Football Casual, when trainers had attained a zenith of importance within U.K. youth culture. I had followed the lead of the older lads of the country, who, since the late 1970s, had been exhibiting signs of extreme obsession toward the once humble training shoe.

An obsessional love of trainers had also started to rear its head in other youth culture 'tribes'. This was the same era where the urban black kids in New York City discovered hip-hop, and turned the sneaker into a 'must-have' essential item in the wardrobe of any self-respecting group member.

The name of this article of footwear may vary depending on where you are in the world, but the love is just the same. Trainers, sneakers, kicks, pumps, plimsolls, runners, gym shoes, whatever name you happen to know them by they have gained a significance that goes way beyond their original sporting intentions. No longer are these shoes confined to the sports field or athletics track. They have been transformed into a culturally significant item of clothing that is capable of producing emotions of love and obsession – even, in some cases, aggression. Unlike the proverbial book and its cover, it *is* possible to judge people by the trainers they wear.

Today, trainers are a ubiquitous item of apparel, worn by everyone – and I mean everyone. Take a look in any closet, from a pensioner's to a child's, and it will contain at least one pair of trainers. Yet even as recent as the early 1970s this was simply not the case. Up until that time, trainers had been mainly worn by sportsmen and women for their original purpose of comfort and to enhance their athletic performance.

Sure, trainers had been worn as a fashion item in the United States by kids in the 1950s, who adopted Converse All Stars as part of their uniform. And in Britain during the 'Swinging '60s, fashion-aware Mods had to be surgically removed from their Spring Courts. The numbers involved, however, were minuscule compared to the mass acceptance of the shoes today.

The intention of this book is to act as a sourcebook, tracing the development of the training shoe from its earliest beginnings. It looks at the technological improvements these shoes underwent, records their cultural appropriation and ends with the present day. It documents the major players in the field as well as looks at the cultural aspects of the rise and rise of the once humble training shoe.

More than anything else, this book is meant as a homage to the trainer. I am certain there will be some mistakes, but despite these I hope I have managed to capture some of the magic. At the end of the day, it's about the shoes.

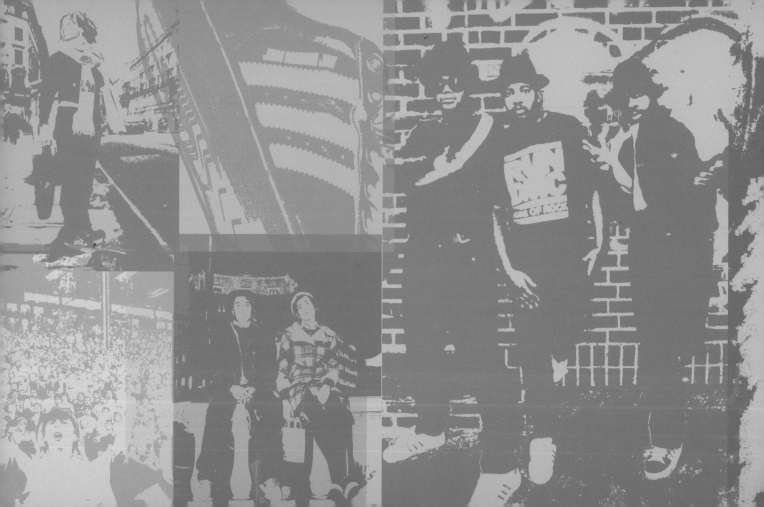

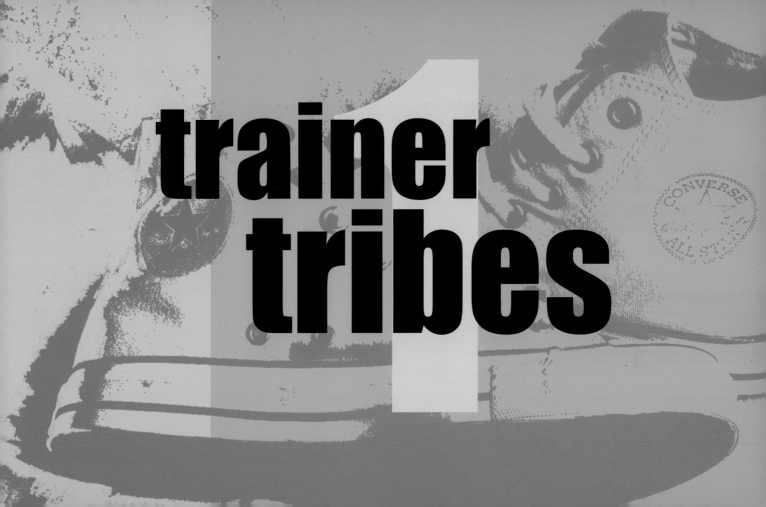

trainer tribes
INTRODUCTION

It's strange that we don't really seem to stop and think that the trainers we all wear are inextricably linked to sport. Before people shout, think about it. Trainers are so popular and so ubiquitous that, almost like an ancient tool from our ancestors, we forget what they are actually designed for.

If you're wearing a pair of adidas Trimm Trab you are being told 'Keep fit'. Try telling 'fashion' posers that their Nike Dunks were named after a basketball move, or are so coloured because they are for an American university basketball team. These shoes are designed for sports and although we wear our trainers everywhere most of us never go near a track or court. They have become the bastion of the streets, dance floors or terraces (bleachers). Even though we all wear sneakers, it is their appropriation by certain youth 'tribes' that makes them the phenomenon they are today.

These tribes constantly adapt the humble sports shoe as a way of making a statement or of belonging. The shoes come in myriad designs and colours – conspicuous branding with connotations of 'tribes' built in. Without the 'tribes' initial use of trainers, they would not be the success they are today in terms of global sales.

Trainer companies owe the tribes a huge 'thank you'.

The next sections on Casuals, Hip-Hop and Skate detail the 'trainer tribes' that have had a particular effect on sneaker sales and development. There are others, such as the L.A.

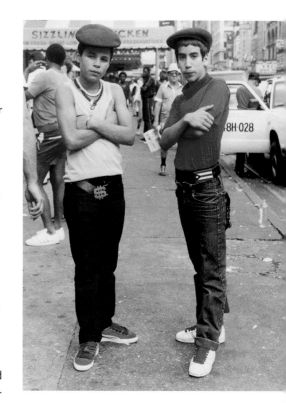

gangs or the initial 1950s kids in the Converse Chucks, but the following three changed the world.

But no matter how important or impressive these three tribes have been, trainer culture is not all about looking back. Things move on and new tribes are constantly striving to invent and be seen, so check out some new tribe members in Street Portraits (*see pages 32–3*), which you can guarantee will be seen on a street near you today.

It is easy to scoff at those who wear trainers outside your 'remit' and become a little too obsessive about the shoes, but I hope you open your eyes, enjoy and 'dig the new breed'.

RIGHT A window display from back in the day.
OPPOSITE It is all a matter of attitude – this was when 'Old Skool' was the 'New Skool'.

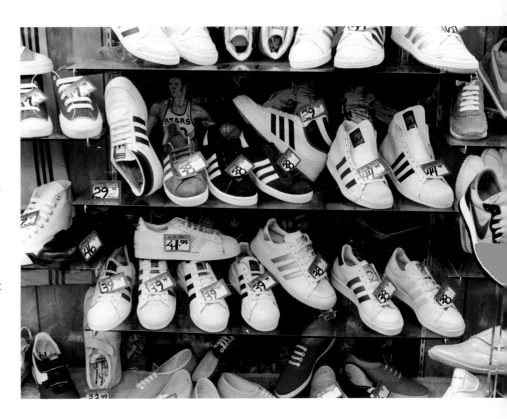

the casuals

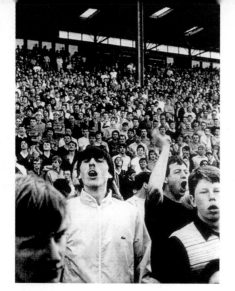

ABOVE Football Casuals in full voice on the football (soccer) terraces.

Some explanation of this, the first entry in our Trainer Tribes chapter, might be necessary, especially for those not living in the U.K. For a nationwide movement that spanned nearly a decade, it's odd that the Casuals is easily the most underground of the tribes and, arguably, the most important in trainer terms.

Somehow the Casuals slipped under the radar of metropolitan-based journalism. As with other urban tribes, it started in working-class areas and, in particular, was linked to the terraces (bleachers) of local football (soccer) teams. It's debatable exactly where in the U.K. the scene first surfaced, but in the late 1970s Liverpool gave birth to 'Scallies', Manchester had its 'Perries' and London had its 'Chaps'. These movements later merged as one definable movement under the umbrella term 'Casuals'.

The Casuals were mainly groups of young men who attached themselves to their local soccer side. The emphasis was on smart and sporting dress in various forms, and a preoccupation with trainer footwear that was obsessional, to say the least.

I hope this manages to blow a hole in the often espoused claim that U.K. trainer culture began only in the late 1980s. I now pass the pen on to those better able to tell the tale. Read on, and welcome to the 'Shock of the Old'.

LONG-HAIRED LOVER (OF ADIDAS) FROM LIVERPOOL
BY JOHN CONNOLLY

Like most fads, wearing trainers as a fashion statement more than likely came about by accident. Let's face it, people have always worn trainers for reasons that have nothing to do with training. Old clips of *Starsky and Hutch*, for example, show Starsky chasing bad guys in adidas Dragons. The 1977 European Cup final in Rome saw Liverpool fans wearing flared Flemings jeans, Levi's tartan shirts and Gola Cobra trainers. Not long after, the terraces of Anfield (Liverpool's football ground) and Goodison Park (Everton's home ground) saw many fans in trousers that were much tighter, granddad shirts and adidas Sambas (or the less expensive Bambas and Mambas). What had started out as an unusual trend soon engulfed the streets of Liverpool.

Most kids probably remember Kicks as their first adidas shoes. But they were not taken seriously by a new wave of fashion-conscious youth. My own first pair of adidas was the classic 1970s' running shoe, TRX. They weren't bought as a fashion item, but actually as running shoes. Then, when I saw older, more clued-up lads in their adidas trainers, they became an essential part of my new wardrobe.

Many of the adidas trainers sported by fellow scousers were 'acquired' on trips to various European countries. Luckily for these travelling fans, most stores then had a policy of leaving shoes in pairs. A lot of the lads were going to Europe and getting hold of trainers that you couldn't

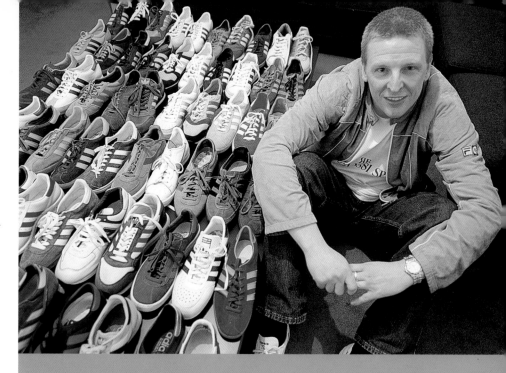

Ex-Football Casual, Kerso, with his amazing collection of training shoes. Kerso, like many trainer fans, is not really a collector – just someone who loves his shoes. The trainers displayed here are typical of the models favoured by the Casuals, such as many adidas City series models, Trimm Trabs and multiple adidas and Diadora models, including the Elite.

find in Liverpool. This started a one-upmanship that didn't escape the attention of a young buyer for adidas based in Liverpool, Robert Wade Smith.

If you were too young (or broke) to visit Europe, one of the best places to get hold of adidas in Liverpool was the sport outlet run by Wade Smith in the Top Man store. After going to the Frankfurt Sports Fair in 1980, Wade Smith wanted the Liverpool branch of Top Man to stock adidas Forest Hills. Adidas insisted on 500 pairs going to its store in Oxford Circus, London, where not a single pair was sold. Although the high price tag was blamed, Wade Smith knew different. He had the unsold stock sent to Liverpool, put them on sale at the beginning of December 1980, and had sold out by Christmas.

After this, he left to set up on his own. Wade Smith was founded in 1982 as a small store selling only adidas shoes. The store probably had the biggest range of adidas shoes in one place anywhere in the world, stocking rare imports from Germany, France, Austria, Switzerland and Holland. Lads still travelled to Europe to acquire trainers, but the opening of Wade Smith managed to quench the thirst of many of these trainer addicts.

Other popular trainers at the time included Puma, with their Argentina and G Vilas shoes; the Diadora Borg Elite was also a cult classic; and Velcro strap-over trainers by Patrick and Donnay were hits. But adidas shoes were still the essential preference due to a few key factors – they had the most extensive range, they were the best made and most importantly they looked the best.

The turn of the 1980s saw more specialized shoes achieve cult Casuals status. Adidas tennis shoes such as Wimbledon, Grand Prix and Grand Slam were essentials. Its specialist running shoes Adistar, Marathon and Oregon were also popular. In fact, adidas had a specialist range for every sport. It produced shoes for obscure sports like handball and skittles. Even the adidas all-weather golf shoe Is Molas were sported by a few. Its casual/leisure trainers proved even more desirable. The likes of Jogger, Jeans and any of their City range were must-haves, as were the phenomenal cult leisure shoes Tenerife, Palermo and Korsica. The adidas Trimm Trab shoe that hit the market in 1982 accounted for 80 per cent of Wade Smith's first-year turnover. Because of the sheer volume sold in Liverpool, nostalgic consumers probably remember the Trimm Trab with the most affection. The shape and sole of the Trimm Trab were duplicated in adidas's new City range.

More stores in the city cashed in on the trend. Stores such as MC Sports, Whittys and Goldrush were doing excellent trade in sports shoes. The emergence of Reebok, New Balance and Nike in the

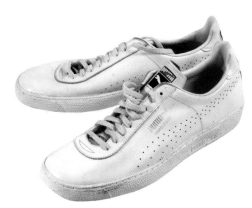

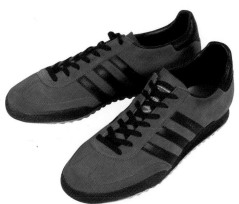

Liverpool trainer domain began. Nike faired better than others and started to gain a foothold with running shoes like Yankee, Intrepid and Internationalist. Its tennis shoes Wimbledon and Bruin also had a decent following in Liverpool. It seems strange now but at the height of trainer popularity, Nike was very much a second-class citizen.

Adidas continued to create the superior trainer and remained most popular in the early to mid 1980s. Columbia, Harvard and Galaxy were light years ahead of the competition. Its running shoes New York, Dallas and Waterproof looked like they were made for astronauts to jog around the Sea of Tranquility. For me, the early ZX range by adidas was probably the last of the brand's great originals. After 1985, the market seemed to be awash with cheap-looking shoes with big plastic

LEFT The famous adidas Jeans and Puma Wimbledon.

tongues, perhaps influenced by a fast-food type of ethic where quality comes second to quantity. Although adidas still made a few reasonable runners, gone was the City range and the new tennis shoes were nothing compared to its early masterpieces. In the late 1980s Reebok tennis and workout shoes became de rigueur with trainer-wearing Liverpudlians.

THE REST OF THE COUNTRY
BY SHAUN SMITH

As three-stripe mania kicked in on Liverpool's Merseyside in the late 1970s, it also gripped their rivals in Manchester, who were trawling foreign fields in search of that rare and – just as importantly – 'easily procured' pair of training shoes.

A small-scale, black economy began to revolve around the demand for designer sportswear and footwear, which spread plague-like across early 1980s' Britain. It mostly revolved around gangs of young men who went to and fought at football games, giving birth to the so-called 'Casuals'. At a time of economic recession in the U.K., the scene was quite literally a two-fingered gesture at everything else occurring in and around the participants' lives. Lads faced with inner-city deprivation, mass youth unemployment or, at best, badly paid jobs simply refused to accept their supposed lot and chose instead to discover the delights of sartorial style.

Spreading like a rash across the country via the bigger city clubs, it reached epidemic proportions. Demand out-stripped supply in both official stockist and black-market arenas and labels such as Lacoste, Fila, Ellesse, Sergio Tacchini and Benetton topped shopping and shoplifting lists. The overall look had rapid, ever-changing, and regional variations, but the one constant was the training shoe. This applied whether you were a 'chirpy Cockney' swaggering up the Holloway Road in Nike Wimbledon and frayed Lois jeans, a 'DLF loon' in an

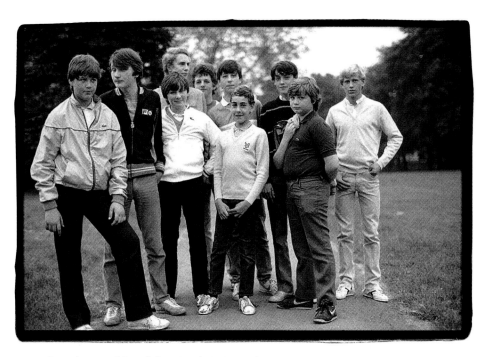

ABOVE An early crew of Casuals from London's East End.

emerald-green Fila Bj and Diadora Borg Elite or a snorkel-clad 'Manc' bowling across the Old Trafford forecourt with semi-flares covering adidas Dublins. Even today, you can spot an old-style soccer head by his general demeanour and choice of footwear.

The trainer worn was, and still is, a give-away to recognizing if someone is really 'right'. Get the trainer wrong and no amount of Stone Island coats or loud housecheck will make you look clued-up. Get it right and you are quite simply right. End of argument.

When it comes to the aesthetics of the training shoe, it might be argued that beauty is in the eye of the beholder? Not true, I'm afraid. Surely it's not that hard to see . . . or is it? Here's a quick test for you. Make a choice between: Puma Sprint or Puma State? Reebok Instapump or Reebok Tennis Classic? Nike Air Max or Nike Internationalist? Adidas Galaxy or adidas Boston? If you chose the first shoe given in each example, then you are likely to be younger than thirty, discovered soccer during the Euro '96 competition and are possibly in need of a visit to your optician. If the second shoe of each pairing was your preferred option, then you are almost certainly older than thirty and still get dewy-eyed when reminiscing about Cerruti 1881 velour tracksuit tops.

Contrary to popular belief, trainer style cannot be bought – no amount of money is enough. You want examples? Noel Gallagher was reportedly spotted buying Acupuncture shoes from Cruise in Glasgow last year – so wrong. TV cook Jamie Oliver in just about any trainers he wears – always wrong. Anyone in anything imported from Japan that is invariably expensive and produced in loud colours – even more wrong. A thirteen-year-old Liverpool lad begging his dad for adidas Kegler Supers last Christmas – most definitely right. And he would not be seen dead wearing Acupuncture shoes either.

As Bing Crosby and Dean Martin famously crooned in *Robin and the Seven Hoods*:

'you've either got or you haven't got style . . .'

RIGHT Adidas Dublins.

the gangs of new york city, hip-hop & sneakers

**WORDS & PHOTOGRAPHS BY
CHARLIE AHEARN**

To those who have been sleeping on Hip-Hop I will try briefly to encapsulate a movement that took a hundred people more than a decade to formulate.

During the 1970s New York City went bankrupt and all civil amenities and social services were cut to the bone. Street gangs marked walls in local neighbourhoods to claim their territory, then individuals began spraying their names on the subways, making the writing masters All City. In the most isolated and impoverished borough, the South Bronx, DJ Kool Herc, wanting to excite his bboy dancers, developed a

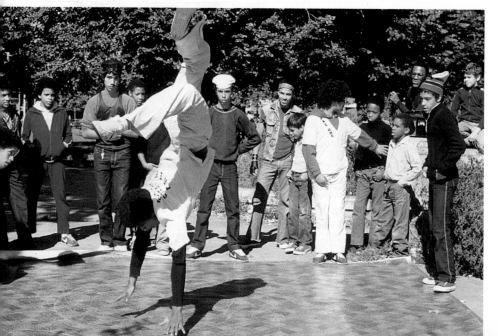

LEFT Frosty Freeze flipping for the Rock Steady Crew – a scene in *Wild Style*.

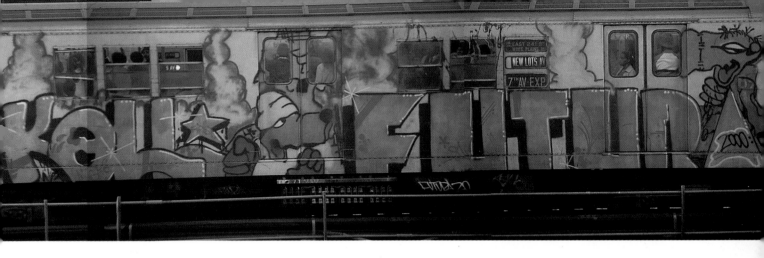

technique in the mid-1970s of looping the drum break of a James Brown record, or other selections, to create a super hot, new percussive sound. DJ Afrika Bambaataa transformed the huge Blade Spades gang into The Mighty Zulu Nation centred around DJ parties and afrocentric cultural events. Grand Master Flash experimented with perfecting his cutting techniques and invited his bboy squad to try flexing their style on the mic, which led to the formation of The Furious MC's. Hip-Hop was born.

Across the Bronx the younger kids jumped into the game. A young bboy turned to the turntables to become DJ Casanova Fly and later one of the greatest MC's as The Grand Master Caz of The Cold Crush Bros. His high-school buddy Prince Whipper Whip learned MC'ing from Caz and then went on to join The Fantastic Five MC's, who were the major street rivals of the Cold Crush. A younger set of kids later sought to revive the forgotten arts of bboying and re-formed The Rock Steady Crew with Crazy Legs,

ABOVE A subway train displaying a complete, eye-popping 'makeover' courtesy of the graffiti legend Futura, in 1981.

Ken Swift, Frosty Freeze and others. Around 1980 I began working with Fab 5 Freddy to document the scene to produce a movie to celebrate Hip-Hop called *Wild Style*. Twenty years later, a similar cast of Hip-Hop pioneers told their story in a photos and flyer book called *Yes Yes Y'all*.

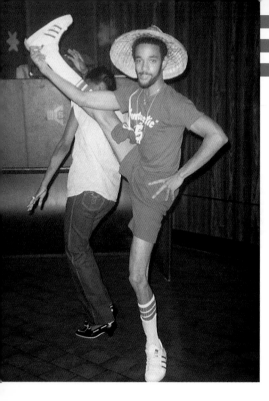

ABOVE Whipper Whip in 1981. Note the Bronx-style socks with stripes matching those on his adidas.

Prince Whipper Whip was one of the original Fantastic Five MC's who rocked the basketball court, the club scene and The Amphitheater in Wild Style. When asked what he was wearing at the time, 'Yo The Fantastic Five always dressed to impress – adidas. I still wear adidas. They tried to come off with their commercial version with the puffy tongue, but now they made them OG (original gangster) with the tongue of leather like before.'

This photograph (*see left*) was taken at The Sparkle, one of the original Kool Herc spots in the Bronx. Whip was going off on the dance floor doing kung fu: 'I always did martial arts. My father was a kung fu instructor. And adidas were perfect for training – light and durable.'

If they are so durable, why do you need so many pairs? Whip laughs: 'Like Nelly says, "once they get stepped on, you got to get a fresh pair".' The other photograph is of Grand Master Caz

(leader of the legendary Cold Crush Bros) going for a shot. The picture was taken on the same court used in the famous basketball scene in *Wild Style*.

Caz remembered that moment: 'I had on my white adidas with green stripes to match my green shirt. I always co-ordinated my outfits like that.'

We were working on *Wild Style* back in the autumn of 1980 and Caz took me up to his bedroom where he lived with his Mom on Creston Boulevard (just two blocks from the basketball court we used in the movie). Caz wanted to show me his two prize collections. First, he spread out a dozen black-and-white marbleized composition books (the kind we all used in grammar school) on the bed, which were crammed with Caz's rhymes all in his incredibly neat handwriting. Caz is one of the greatest lyricists in Hip-Hop and this was the proof.

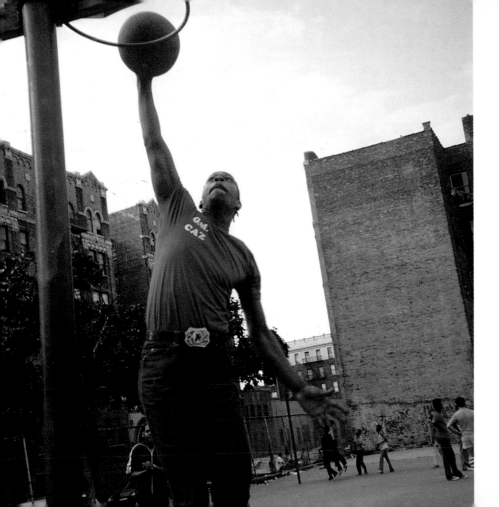

Then he opened his closet door to reveal a floor-to-ceiling stack of sneaker boxes, all in mint condition, all Pumas and adidas. Out came the boxes, lovingly opened on the bed and displayed like jewels. Mostly they were white shell-toed adidas. 'I never did black.' Not one trainer showed any signs of wear.

'When I was young, I went to Catholic school,' Caz explained, 'and we had to wear shoes every day. Every day! We had to wear shoes to gym class! So when I got loose it was sneakers and I been a sneaker pimp ever since.'

LEFT One of the earliest of the Hip-Hop DJs, Grand Master Caz, in action on the court.

my adidas & me
ADIDAS & RUN DMC

As we know, the Hip-Hop movement had deep associations with trainers from its very beginnings. However, it was one band that really became associated with a love for adidas sneakers. That band was Run DMC. By no means was DMC the only one of the Hip-Hop circle to embrace sneaker culture, but they were the first to really openly declare their love through music. DMC had both a substantial and long-lasting effect on youth culture, but almost more importantly it was DMC that made the corporate brands aware of the sheer scope of the affection urban youth had for their trainers.

Run DMC can be attributed with causing a seismic change in the annals of trainer brand history by becoming the first non-athletes ever sponsored by a sports company. DMC had long exhibited the Hip-Hop obsession with their footwear and felt strongly enough to write a song declaring this love to the world. The single *My adidas* went on to be a commercial hit and awoke something within the sleeping corporate giant of adidas.

A decision that would seem obvious today was more difficult back then. The question of whether hardcore rappers were appropriate for adidas endorsees almost split the company. Something had to give, so a team of adidas employees were persuaded to watch the band in action. They eventually found themselves in the unusual situation of attending a Run DMC concert – to be precise, it was the Philadelphia date on the band's Raising Hell tour, which they shared with the Beastie Boys.

RIGHT *My adidas;* Run DMC sports their brand of choice when it comes to footwear.

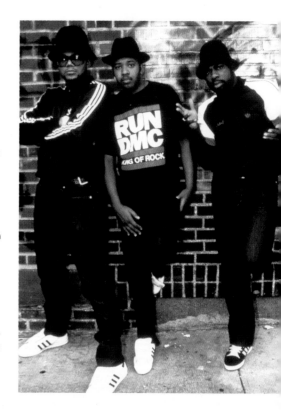

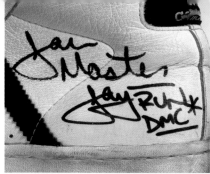

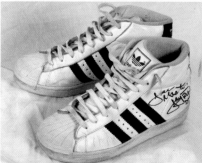

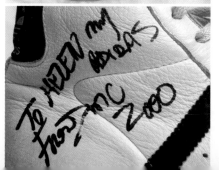

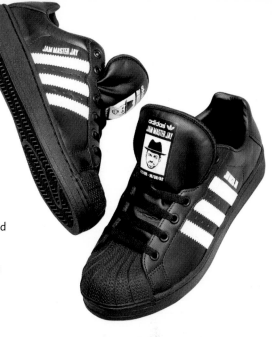

In one simple act, Run DMC had made up the mind of the German invitees. Before playing their latest single, Run DMC commanded their audience: 'Everybody wearing adidas wave your sneakers in the air!' To the astonishment of the adidas corporate guests, most of the 25,000-strong audience complied.

The adidas company immediately agreed to sponsor the group and even began custom-making stage clothes for the band members, who went on to launch the now legendary black leather Run DMC tracksuits. The following year adidas's U.S. profits were boosted by some $35 million.

However, it is not for commercial reasons alone that Run DMC will always be associated with sneakers. In speaking of their own genuine love, DMC found a voice that spoke for a whole generation.

ABOVE Limited edition adidas shell-toes were released in homage to the late Jam Master Jay and have his face imprinted on the tongue. **LEFT** Adidas Pro-Models, signed by the band's late Jam Master Jay.

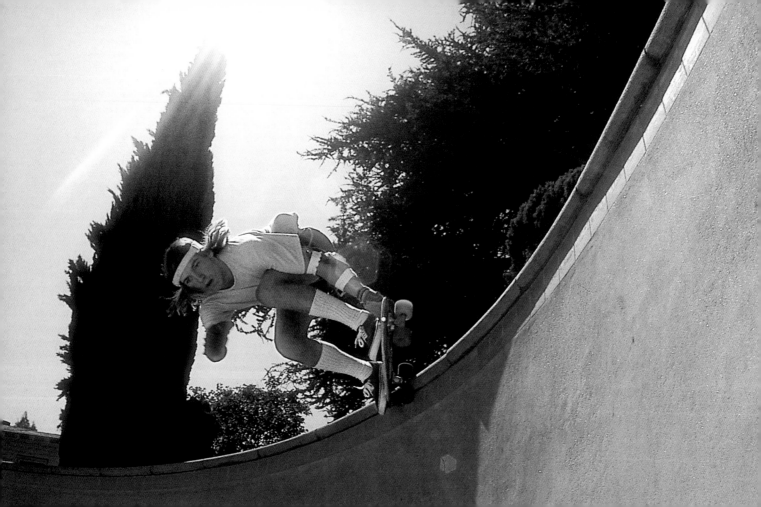

the skate story

AARON HAWKINS

Skateboarding is an individualistic, athletic art form. Inspired by style and the release of radical energy, mostly present during the rebellious adolescent years and in those who never lose that spark, skateboarders by their very nature are the present-day, concrete-jungle urban guerrillas. They *need* good shoes to survive.

In the early 1970s Vans 'deck' shoes were only $6 a pair and, by the nature of their sport, skateboarders went through a lot of them. And not only Vans, there were also Sperry Top Siders, Converse Jack Purcells and Chuck Taylors and Keds casual sneakers. They really worked their shoes over and needed to buy replacements every several weeks or so. Their short street life made the cost of shoes almost as important as their grip. Vans was a small 'mom and pop' company at this time, manufacturing all of its products in a tiny factory in southern California. You could buy them only from a select few Vans storefronts that were spread around the area.

For just $1 extra you could customize your 'deck' shoe fabrics, and you could also choose the colours you wanted. Original Z-Boy Wentzle Ruml was one of the first ever to specify his own two-tone colour style, especially the navy-and-red combination. They were an instant hit on the west side of L.A. with the Dogtown crew and their followers. It was the cool thing to do, go to the Vans store for custom-made Vans.

OPPOSITE Paul Constantineua rocking his two-toned Vans at the famous Dog Bowl, photographed in 1976.

Fellow Z-Boy Tony Alva was becoming world famous by this time, so when pictures of him wearing Vans began to pop up in *Skateboarder* magazine, needless to say Vans benefited greatly from it. Many of the other Dogtown skaters, along with various other skate pros at the time, would wear custom-coloured Vans almost exclusively.

Eventually Vans got together with the more professionally orientated Z-Boy Stacy Peralta, who helped to design a shoe Vans made specifically *for* skaters. This was a step in the right direction, but the company spoiled a good thing by suddenly more than tripling shoe prices from their original $7 price tag. They skated good, though, and were sold in their tens of thousands. Skateboarding was hitting its biggest boom to date, but at that higher price kids realized if they were going to be spending that type of money then they might as well start looking at the other brands that were

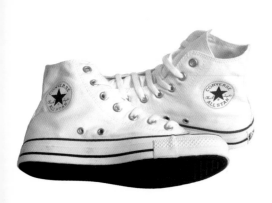

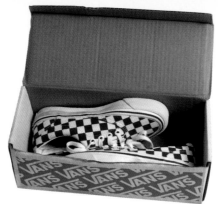

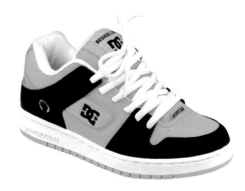

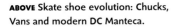

ABOVE Skate shoe evolution: Chucks, Vans and modern DC Manteca.

already priced at that level, such as Nike. Seeing the potential, Nike started to give Alva some of its earliest Blazers. And those, along with other heavily padded ankle basketball shoes, became popular for those with dough in the know.

However, the bulk of the expanding vertical-ramp and skatepark population stayed true to their Converse Chuck Taylors and their even flashier Vans models, favouring Vans with the chequerboard

lo-tops and aqua-panelled hi-tops and Converse with bleached logos and tags on its classic uppers. The outsoles proved to be extra grippy and flexible, which made them perfect for the style of skating that was going down at the time.

With tricks such as 'rock-n-rolls', 'smith grinds' and 'laybacks' there was a need for upper foot/ankle mobility with a glue-footed stance. The problem now was that the midsoles were too firm and provided minimal heel cushioning. In addition, the canvas side panels got ripped to pieces in a matter of days. There wasn't a skater

alive at that time who didn't use strategically placed Shoe-Goo and duct tape. Some people took these repairs to a whole new style level by sewing patches of fabric over the holes, so that each shoe had its own unique look. But when the street-skating revolution started to emerge in 1985, everything began to change.

Frustrated and tired of bruised heels and shredded toes, skaters started to look at early model Nike and adidas basketball shoes as viable options to skate in. After all, the leather side panels were far more robust than the canvas ones found on the Vans/Converse shoes, and basketball shoes had the better insole/midsole/outsole cushioning and ankle support needed for high-impact court landings. Ankle support was believed to be essential for preventing injury while trying those first 'kickflips' and '360 shove-its'. The outsole's grip was nowhere near the same as the Converse and Vans, however, but the new comfort pluses seemed to outweigh the minuses. Of course, having street skating's master innovator Mark Gonzales rocking the Air Jordan 1s (which, it is believed, he purchased at a closing-down sale because they were cheap) certainly helped. The 'Gonz' was God and everything he did was copied by everyone, in much the same way as Alva influenced the previous generation.

Many professional skaters followed suit, and soon kids across the globe were scrambling for any kind of hi-top basketball shoe they could find. Basketball shoes became the *only* choice for the younger kids during the late 1980s. Adidas, Nike, Troop, British Knights and even Reeboks were at the forefront of hi-top skate and bboy fashion, with some small following of people using the Puma and Pony lo-tops at the local street-skating spot.

The brands' accessibility spawned a new approach to skate shoes from this point on. Vision Street Wear produced a version of the Air Force 1 hi-top, and a new upstart brand, Airwalk, walked down that bulky support road as well. It was a significant departure from the 'old-skool' Vans' approach, but skating was evolving and so were the shoes. Though seemingly insignificant at the time, you can look

RIGHT Recently released skate shoes from Gonzales.

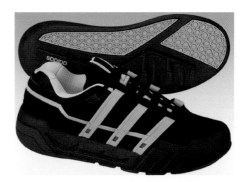

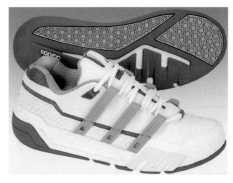

back and see the massive effects these brands have had in shaping the course of shoe-design culture. They opened a lot of people's eyes to the possibilities, merging the worlds of fashion and function for the first time. Ultimately, however, a lack of direction lead to their fall from popularity, and eventually motivated a few business-minded skaters to start their own brands. After all, only skaters could relate to other skaters when it came to balancing limited funds and good product development.

Etnies (Sole Technologies and its expanding family of speciality footwear brands) came first with the 'skater owned and operated' approach to marketing, releasing the Natas Kaupas signature shoe (the first pro-model shoe of this next generation). The launch was very successful with the cooler skate shops, and the brand enjoyed a steady boom of growth for the first few years. Soon after, other brands such as Duffs, Dukes,

Simple and DC picked up on the momentum out there and created their own styled-brand approach. DC Shoes, in particular (named after the initials of Droors Clothing), began in the early 1990s, featuring the personalities of top pros Danny Way and Colin McKay. DC immediately gained considerable market share through its technically advanced shoe designs and high-powered print marketing. Together with Etnies, DC placed major pressure on the then giant Airwalk brand to perform better as a skater-proven shoe company. Its designs had become disconnected from the underground, and had drifted further and further away from their origins in the skateboarding world. Challenged, Airwalk seemingly turned tail and ran to the nearest Foot Locker for sales direction, soon plummeting into a downward spiral as a result. By now, the 'skater-owned' brands had staked their claim in the shoe world and the whole game would never be the same again.

The movement of skateboarder-driven shoe companies pushing the envelope has continued to grow in numbers right up to this day. Retail skate shops depend on the high profit margins from shoe sales to pay the bills. Major multisport footwear companies look to the skate industry for inspiration and ideas (and vice versa). Total annual skate-shoe sales run into hundreds of millions of dollars, and many skater-owned companies have profited from these successes – so much so that some professional skateboarders can afford to buy legitimate mansions just from their pro-model shoe royalties alone. The current situation is a pretty far-fetched reality compared with the days of $7 custom Vans, duct tape and Shoe-Goo.

RIGHT Skater Shogo Kubo wearing early Nike hi-tops in 1977.

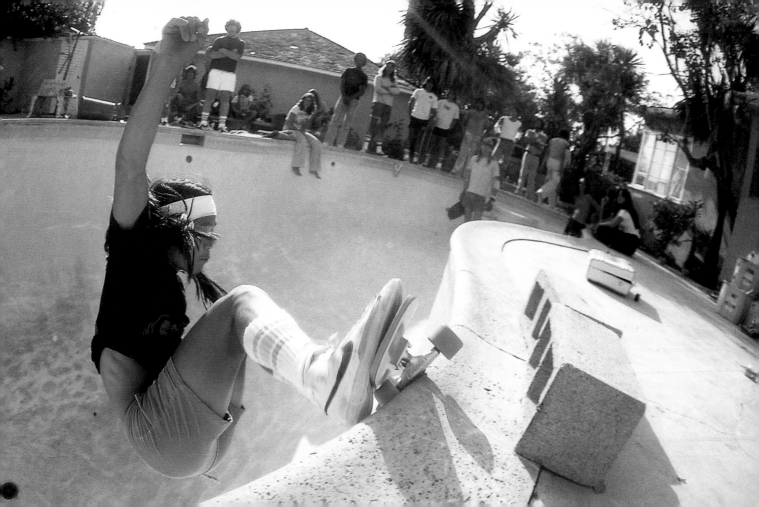

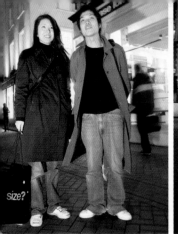
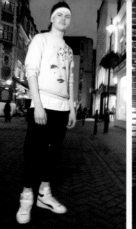
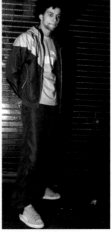
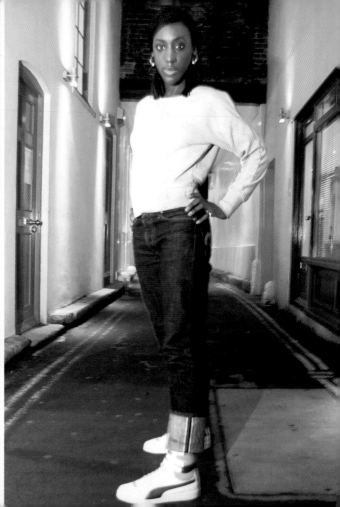

street portraits

SOME OF THE **NEW BREEDS** OF TRAINER FANS ON A STREET NEAR YOU

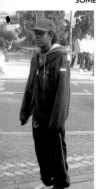
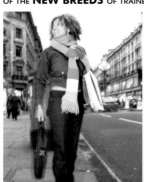
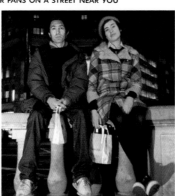

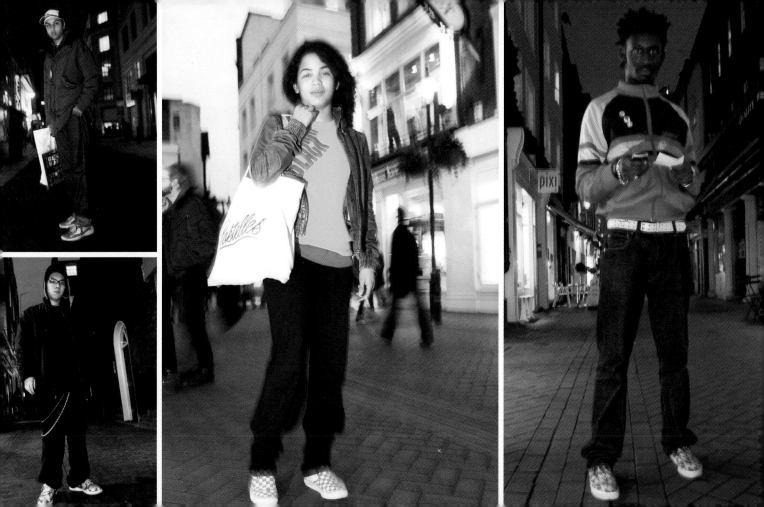

hall of fame 2

hall of fame
INTRODUCTION

To quote the late, great Bob Marley:

**If you know your history,
then you will know where
I'm coming from.**

To understand how we've arrived at this particular point in trainer development it's important to have some understanding of trainer history. To help in this, it seems logical to create a trainer 'Hall of Fame'.

This should be no 'personal taste' Hall of Fame, but a chronological listing of those training shoes that have had more of a pronounced influence on trainer development than others. Before being bombarded with irate demands about why I omitted this or that favourite shoe, I must point out that this is not my own, or any other individual's, list of favourite shoes (my personal list, for example, would contain only three of those below).

Rather, this is an attempt to draw up a definitive list of truly significant shoes.

The prerequisite for a trainer's entry into this hallowed Hall Of Fame is that the shoe must have been groundbreaking in some major way – either technically or aesthetically – and so have influenced the course of trainer development. However, there are a special few included that have gained entry purely because they have had such a pronounced cultural effect, proving so enduringly popular that they have become a part of trainer folklore.

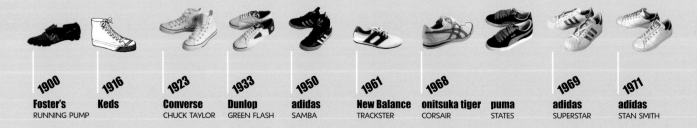

1900
Foster's
RUNNING PUMP

1916
Keds

1923
Converse
CHUCK TAYLOR

1933
Dunlop
GREEN FLASH

1950
adidas
SAMBA

1961
New Balance
TRACKSTER

1968
onitsuka tiger
CORSAIR

puma
STATES

1969
adidas
SUPERSTAR

1971
adidas
STAN SMITH

The initial entries into the list are embroiled in claim and counterclaim for the 'ownership' or 'invention' of trainers themselves. In particular there is an on-going Anglo-American disagreement, between the Goodyear and Dunlop companies on this point.

To reiterate, this Hall of Fame is not one that is made up of my own personal taste in sneakers. However, just for interest, or as a bit of background, or perhaps just to cause some debate, my own top 10 list would be something like this:

1   adidas ZX250

2   Nike Air Max 90 (black/red)

3   adidas Trimm Trab

4   adidas ZX500

5   Nike Wimbledon

6   adidas Stan Smith

7   Nike Air Max 1

8   Puma State

9   Nike Air Max 95 (grey/green only)

10 Nike Hawaii

At the end of this chapter we can then look at the training shoes that have been made famous by the stars of stage and screen, as well as those that have been endorsed by the giants of the sporting world.

So, ladies and gentlemen, come with me on a trip through time. To find our first entries in our trainer Hall of Fame, we really have to dig deep into the annals of trainer archaeology. Indeed, we have to go back to that mist-shrouded time before trainers even existed. . .

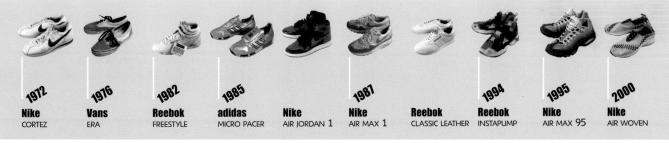

1972
Nike
CORTEZ

1976
Vans
ERA

1982
Reebok
FREESTYLE

1985
adidas
MICRO PACER

Nike
AIR JORDAN 1

1987
Nike
AIR MAX 1

Reebok
CLASSIC LEATHER

1994
Reebok
INSTAPUMP

1995
Nike
AIR MAX 95

2000
Nike
AIR WOVEN

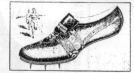

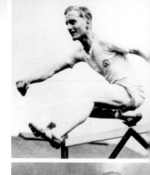

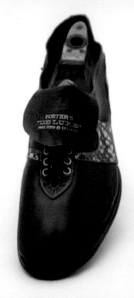

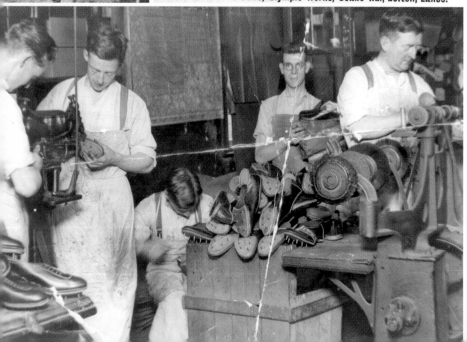

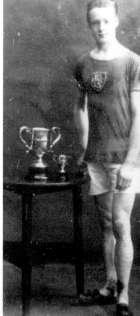

foster's
RUNNING PUMP

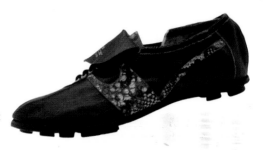

If I could include sound effects I would insert them here. But I can't, so instead imagine all the time-flying image clichés you can muster – swirling mist, hyper-fast ticking clocks, calendars turning themselves backward and so on. You've got it. We are, rather contentiously, going to try and start with the first of the first.

This issue could rage back and forth and is mainly fought either side of the Atlantic. Claim is mixed in with counterclaim for all manner of 'firsts' in the world of trainers. 'We were the first to use vulcanization,' comes the cry. 'No, we were,' is the inevitable retort. 'Ah! But we had the first rubber-soled shoes. . .' And so on.

Although there were various developments in the use of bonding rubber to canvas throughout the late nineteenth century, and these 'plimsolls' were utilized for 'leisure wear', not many of these shoes were actually produced for sports. Although Dunlop and Converse were undoubtedly involved in initial trainer development, it was not until 1917 that Converse developed their basketball shoe, the All Star, and Dunlop was not even a sporting brand until 1928. However, one company that is still in existence today as a major sporting brand developed the Running Pump.

That company is now known as Reebok, but it was way back in 1895 that a certain Joseph William Foster, a runner living in Bolton, in the north of England, developed running spikes for fellow athletes. By 1904, he was selling his 'Foster's Running Spike' to a worldwide athletic market. But it was sometime around 1905 or 1906 that Foster developed his 'Foster's Running Pumps' designed for athletes who ran on roads and, rather strangely, wrestled. These very early 'pumps' can arguably be claimed to be the first trainers/sneakers/pumps of all time.

A new industry was born, and the entrepreneurial Foster marketed the running pumps with remarkable zeal, and so the company grew. Initially developed under the guise of J. W. Foster and Sons, eventually, in 1958, the control of the family business was taken up by Foster's grandsons, and the brand we know today as Reebok was launched on the world.

keds

If you want shoes with lots of pep, get Keds. For bounce and zoom in every step, get Keds.

It was in 1917 that Keds, supported by this dubiously 'catchy' advertising slogan, were released in the United States.

Behind the introduction of Keds, lies a tale of two protagonists who were to effect the world of footwear forever. The story begins back in 1862, when Charles

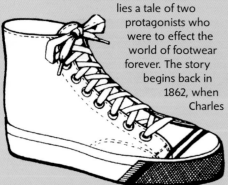

Goodyear (of today's famous Goodyear Tyre fame) patented the process known as 'vulcanization' in order to create industrial rubber.

The story moves on to 1892, when the U.S. Rubber Company began producing (using Goodyear's techniques) rubber specifically to be used for the soles of shoes. These canvas shoes with rubber soles became known as 'croquet shoes', after their use by players of that genteel sport. However, U.S. Rubber comprises up to 30 assorted smaller companies, some producing these shoes under a variety of names.

It is in 1916 that the two stories converge, when Goodyear and U.S. Rubber merged to form a new company. With the demand for rubber-soled footwear increasing, the company decide to produce an entirely new rubber-soled shoe. But what to call it? Initially the name was going to be Peds (from the Latin meaning 'foot'). But fate intervened, and it turned out that this name was already held as a trademark. The choice then narrowed and came down to either Veds or Keds. Thankfully, in a decision that avoided any future *Star Trek* connotations, Keds came out on top.

Keds were not only an early form of sports shoe, they also helped popularize the term 'sneakers'. This came about when the advertising firm behind Keds decided to appropriate the term that had been used in the late nineteenth century (describing quiet, rubber-soled shoes) in order to increase product awareness of Keds.

The company grew and in 1949 Keds launched a line of shoes aimed principally at the basketball market. This specialized line of footwear was known as Pro-Keds, and it is by this name that we know the company to this day.

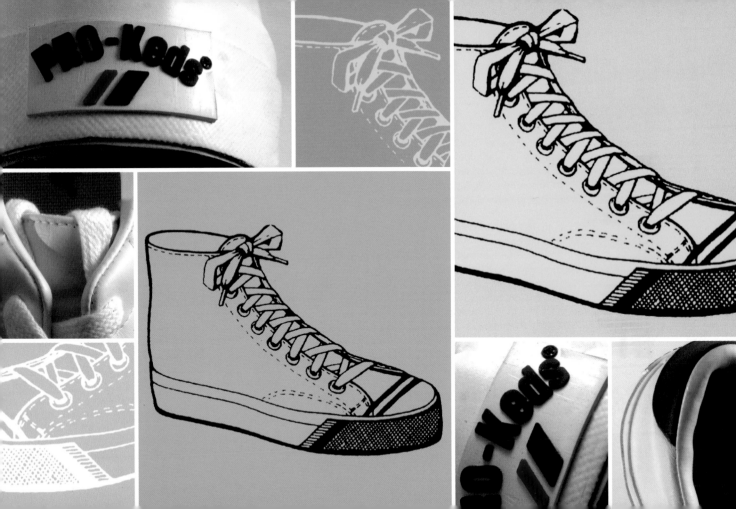

converse all star

CHUCK TAYLOR

The Converse All Star: what more is there to say about a living legend? Hardly changed in construction and appearance since being unleashed on a growing basketball-interested public in 1917 by the Converse Rubber Corporation, it is the oldest sneaker still in production today, as well as the best-selling sneaker of all time.

Initially available only in black, the All Star didn't really take off. However, four years later Charles H. Taylor, a basketball player with the Akron Firestones, joined the Converse sales team. Taylor travelled the country hosting basketball clinics, after which he would sell All Stars to aspiring stars. By 1923 'Chuck' Taylor had been so successful that he was consulted about modifications to the shoe. On his advice, greater ankle support and increased traction were incorporated. More importantly, in what was the first case of athletic endorsement, the name Chuck Taylor was added to the ankle patch. Taylor went on to become the official fitness consultant for the entire U.S. armed forces, but before that he made what must have been one of the worst business decisions ever. When offered a royalty on every shoe sold, he opted instead for his favoured bonus – a new car every year. Since then, millions of pairs have been sold.

Due to demand, off-white 'Chucks' (as they were known) were introduced. After years of basketball teams dying their off-whites in team colours, Converse eventually reacted to demand and, in 1966, produced new colours. By 1968, Converse had 80 per cent of the sneaker industry, and Chuck Taylor was inducted into the basketball Hall of Fame.

Chucks are now seen in myriad colours and patterns and have appeared in more than 100 films. Around 30,000 pairs are sold each day worldwide and by 1997 over 550 million pairs had been sold. The design never seems to go away. Picked up by skaters and New York new wave, among others, Chucks always seem to have a following somewhere in the world.

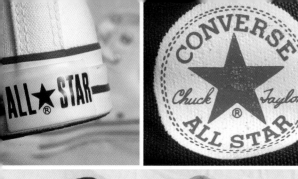
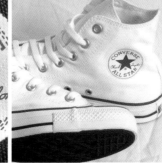
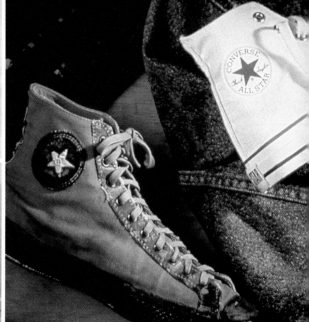
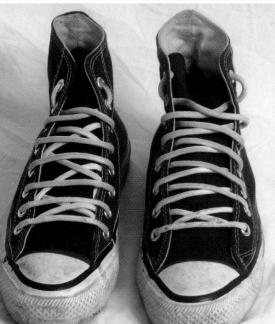
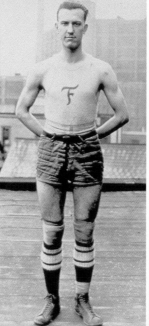
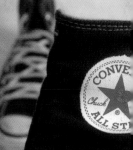
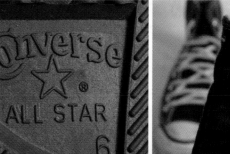

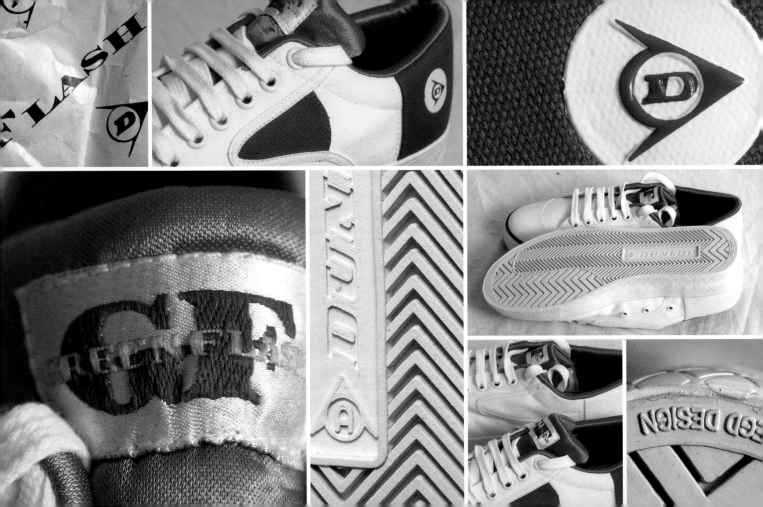

dunlop
GREEN FLASH

Everything needs a beginning, and I suppose we could say that it all started back in Britain in the 1830s. This was when a certain John Boyd Dunlop discovered how to bond canvas to rubber. In the 1890s, Dunlop's Liverpool Rubber Company started to develop sports shoes, known as 'sand shoes', so named because they were worn at the beach by Victorian vacationers.

It is from these shoes that the term plimsoll was applied to sports shoes, as the point at which the canvas and rubber was bonded supposedly looked like the Plimsoll line found on ships' hulls. These Dunlop plimsolls became all-purpose gym shoes during the early years of the twentieth century, but 1933 saw the introduction of the shoe that would go on to become a design classic – the Dunlop Green Flash 1555. This shoe had higher-quality canvas and incorporated a herringbone pattern on the sole for better grip on the tennis court. It went on to become one of the biggest selling sports shoes of all time and is still made today.

The great British tennis player Fred Perry was Green Flash clad when he went on to win Wimbledon three times in succession from 1934. From this point on, the legend grew. Dunlop has sold more than 25 million pairs, with a million a year being sold in the U.K. alone at the height of their popularity.

With the advance of trainer technology and fashion, Green Flash lost some street credibility. However, form is temporary, class is permanent. Times have gone full circle, and Green Flash is enjoying its moment in the sun once more. Dunlop even hooked up with young fashion firms, such as YMC, to give the design a make-over.

In the high profile world of fashion and sport, few styles bear the test of time; even fewer become design icons. The Dunlop Green Flash lays claim to both.

adidas
SAMBA

The adidas Samba is included in this Hall of Fame since it is the granddaddy of adidas shoes. It holds two records for adidas: it is not only the company's biggest selling shoe of all time, it is also the longest running model still in production.

If ever a shoe could be called 'old skool' this is it, and quite literally, too. The Samba is usually the first trainer that many people remember owning. It was the shoe that your mother bought you at about seven years of age to knock about in the schoolyard playing soccer. Later on, it did have a fashion following among those who were into simple, classic design, but this is probably the one shoe in the Hall of Fame that is still primarily used for its original sporting intentions.

Although the Dassler brothers had been producing sports shoes since the 1920s, it was not until their acrimonious split in 1948 that Adolph and his brother Rudolph went their separate ways and adidas was formed. This fascinating story has the plot a good soap scriptwriter would die for, and is told elsewhere in the book (*see pages 90–3*). However, to summarize here, Rudolph went on to form Puma, while Adolph formed adidas.

This bit of background is retold here in order to give historical perspective to a shoe that is still in production today. Adolph had long geared his sports-shoe production to meet the demands of the people who would utilize the shoe itself. Being a keen soccer player, he had many contacts within the sporting world. Thus, it was in 1950 that adidas produced the Samba, and although the shoe is now commonly included as part of an indoor soccer kit, it was initially made to give better traction for those playing on ice, snow and frozen ground.

The shoe is made with full-grain kangaroo leather with a reinforced suede trim. The toe cap has extra strengthening to give added protection when kicking the ball. But it is not for these facts alone that we respect the Samba – this shoe is a classic.

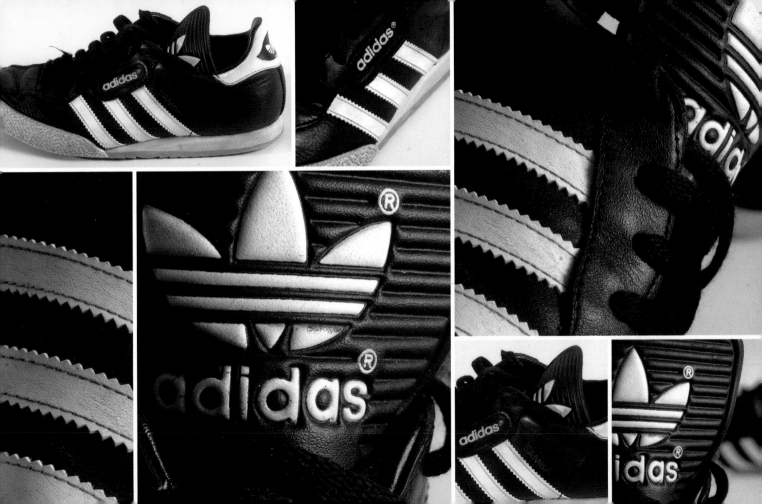

new balance
TRACKSTER

A Massachusetts-based company, New Balance started in the early 1900s, but in those years it had been mainly involved in orthopaedic shoe development, concentrating on arch supports to give wearers 'New Balance'. Up until 1961 it had made only small forays into the running world, but the state capital, Boston, was fast becoming a major base for marathon running and athletics in general.

After a few attempts the company finally produced the model that not only launched the company onto the sports shoe market, but also left an indelible mark on training shoe development. This model was the New Balance Trackster. Two major features really made it stand out. First, the Trackster was the world's first performance running shoe made with a rippled rubber sole (later adopted by many other companies). Second, it was the first model to feature 'width fitting'. This feature is seen by those at the company as its major unique selling point.

Width fitting means that the shoe is available in a range of different widths, using a sizing system that starts from a narrow '2A' and goes up to an extra-wide '4E'. To this day company representatives constantly measure people's feet at race events throughout the world and have discovered that more than 50 per cent of participants require non-standard width fittings.

However, the Trackster is also unique in New Balance terms, as it is one of the only models produced by the company that does not use its unique numbering system to differentiate the various models.

This groundbreaking shoe is being relaunched worldwide in selected outlets in 2003 as a tribute to the importance of its unique features.

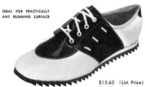
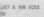

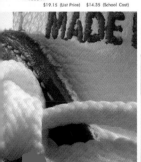

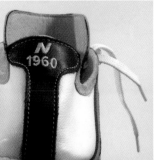

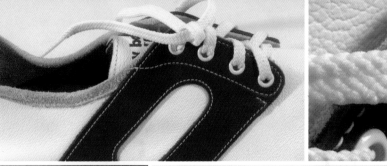

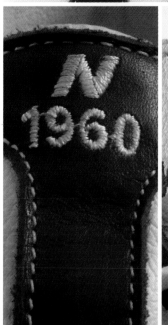

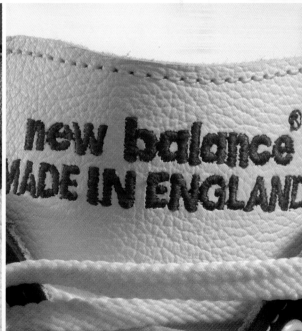

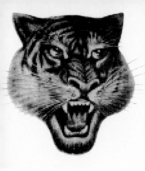
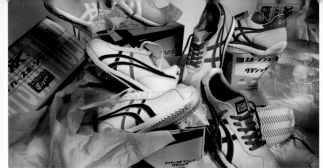
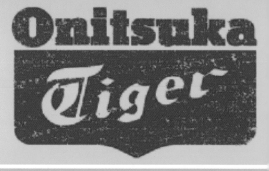
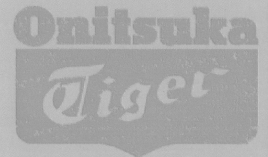
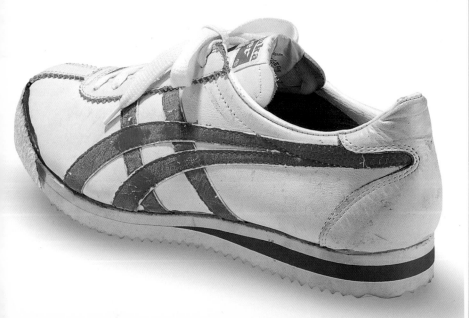

onitsuka tiger
CORSAIR

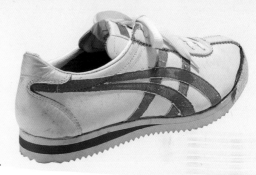

The training shoe company Onitsuka was the forerunner of the brand we know today as Asics. Founded in Kobe, Japan, in 1949 by Kihachiro Onitsuka, the brand became known as Onitsuka Tiger because the early shoes carried a tiger logo on the arch of the foot. Later on the tiger stripes were added to the sides of the shoes.

Onitsuka earns an entry in the Hall of Fame for a number of reasons, not least due to the early technical developments found in the shoe, and also because Onitsuka played a major part in the development of Nike.

The company entered the world of training shoes in 1949 when Kihachiro Onitsuka, acting on his belief that playing sports was the best way to rehabilitate juvenile delinquents, endeavoured to make the best sports shoes he could. Using ideas from the world around him, Onitsuka pioneered new methods in trainer production. For example, by observing a local species of octopus he had the idea of sunken soles to help grip. Another development was the adaptation of a motorcycle air-cooling system to cool the feet of runners. The result was the Onitsuka Magic Runner.

In 1963 these high-tech, low-priced Onitsuka athletic shoes were imported into the United States through a pair of entrepreneurs, Phil Knight and Bill Bowerman. At this time they were operating as Blue Ribbon Sports (BRS), but later became the co-founders of Nike. After initial successes with sales, BRS became involved with Onitsuka in the design of the shoes, developing the Marathon and Boston models for the company.

One of the shoes that Bowerman worked on was the Onitsuka Tiger Corsair. After Bowerman redesigned the shoe, it was manufactured in Japan to his specifications and became the Onitsuka Tiger Cortez, and was a major seller for the Japanese company in 1968. In order to identify the very rare version of the Onitsuka Cortez model, look for the 'Mexico T-24' label (meaning 24 hours training resistible).

The two operations later split and and in 1972 the American duo went totally alone and formed Nike. The Cortez name was kept by Nike and became the now famous Nike Cortez (*see pages 58–9*).

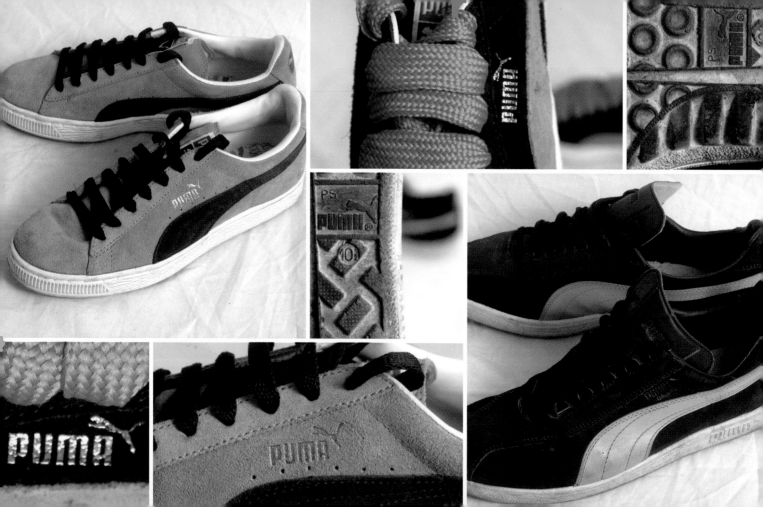

puma
SUEDE/STATE

The Puma Suede, also known as Puma State, is probably the most instantly recognizable of all the entries in the listing of 'grand old brands'. There is nothing particularly groundbreaking about this sneaker, but it would be impossible to develop a Hall of Fame without its inclusion. Equally loved by various trainer faithfuls, the Suede has even been involved in historical matters on a global scale. At the 1968 Olympics, the shoe (released the same year) was worn by Tommy Smith, the prominent equal-rights activist athlete, when he made his famous Black Power salute (*see also page 202*).

The Suedes gained greater prominence in 1974 when they were worn and endorsed by the 'Michael Jordan' of the 1970s, Walt 'Clyde' Frazier of the New York Knicks. The Frazier-endorsed shoe became known as the Puma Clyde. The Clydes instantly became a hit as Frazier was known not only for his basketball skills, but also for being sharp dressed and smooth with the ladies off the court. Clyde Frazier was a man who had style and his trademark was wearing a different-coloured Clyde on each foot. At one point in 1985 more than 2 million pairs of the Clyde were sold in the United States alone.

In cultural terms the Suede can be credited as the first shoe of bboyism. The shoe was made famous by Hip-Hop crews, such as the New York City Breakers and the Rock Steady Crew, who wore them constantly at early Hip-Hop jams in New York City (*see pages 20–5*).

The sneaker's cult status continued even after Hip-Hop's golden years. When the Beastie Boys bounced on stage during their 'Check Your Head' tour in 1994 wearing blue Suedes, almost instantly fans were clamouring for the shoes with the sign of the leaping cat.

Call it what you will, the Suede/State/Clyde is an integral part of training shoe history, and the Puma shoe is a timeless piece of classic design.

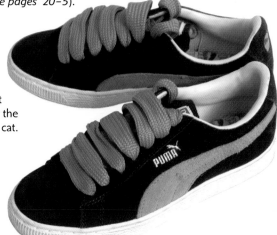

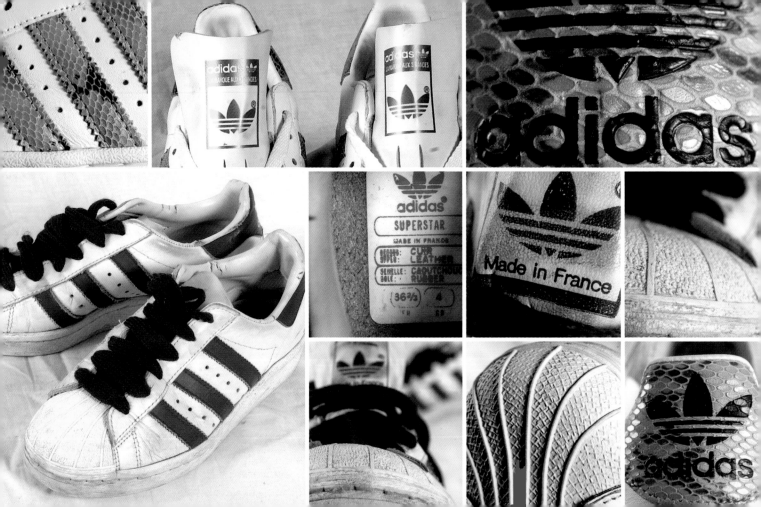

adidas

SUPERSTAR

Say the term 'old skool' to anyone and probably the first sneakers that spring to mind are the adidas Superstar, which, arguably, could be termed the classic of all classics. How else do you explain the fact that a training shoe first introduced in 1969 was still the biggest-selling shoe globally in 2001?

Even though the Superstar was the first low-top basketball shoe to feature an all-leather upper, it is not for its technological features that it enters the Hall of Fame. This shoe's inclusion can be attributed to the cultural effect it has had throughout the world. Basically, the Superstar can be seen every day, everywhere around the globe – in all types of places and on all kinds of feet.

The feature that gave the shoe its famous nickname, the rubber 'shell toe', was developed as a means of protecting the toes of basketball players. The rubber cap did give protection and stability, but the moulding also resembled the outside of a shell, and so the nickname was born. Legend has it the initial request for the design came from the one and only Kareem Abdul Jabbar, who wore the shoes on their release. He had requested the development of a lo-top basketball shoe in order to gain extra agility around the court. However, the Superstar also came in a hi-top version and, thus, the adidas Pro-model was born (even though the shell toe was half suede at first).

The model was so popular that it became standard prison issue in the United States, a fact that added to the shell-toe legend. The shoe grew even more popular with the advent of Hip-Hop in late 1970s' New York, when the local bboys and fly girls sported the shoes as part of their new look. However, the shoes really went 'boom' when they were picked up by Run DMC, who even wrote the song *My adidas* in homage to their Ultra Stars. To this day, Superstars are associated with chunky laces or none at all, and are an essential part of the urban wardrobe.

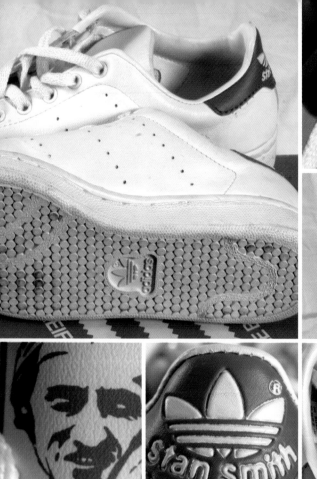
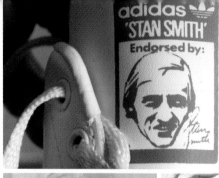

adidas
'STAN SMITH'
Endorsed by:

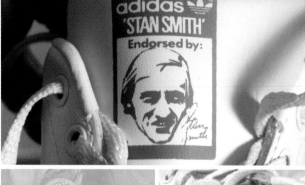

adidas
STAN SMITH
dorsed b

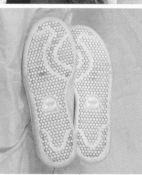

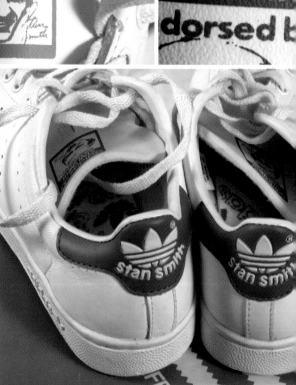

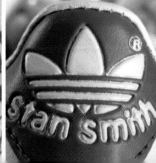

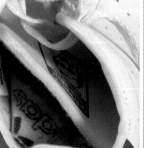
stan smith

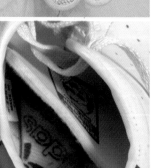

adidas

STAN SMITH

Sometimes less is more, and this is certainly the case with the adidas Stan Smith. This is another entry that has been included in the Hall of Fame due to the enduring quality of the design and the long-lasting effect it has had on trainer design and culture. Some shoes are popular in one country and not another, but the shoe we know as the Stan Smith is one of the few designs that you will see in every city in the world.

Introduced way back in 1965, the sneaker was unique as the first all-leather performance tennis shoe. However, the shoe was also unique visually. Instead of the usual external three adidas stripes, there are three rows of perforations through the leather upper.

However, the shoe did not always exhibit Stan Smith's famous face on the tongue of the shoe. When first introduced the model was originally endorsed by a lesser-known French tennis player, Robet Haillet. Then, it was Mr Haillett's name on the tongue. History took another turn when, in 1971, the shoes were endorsed and renamed after an American, the recent U.S. Open winner Stan Smith.

Since then it has gone on to be one of the best-selling shoes of all time, having sold more than 30 million pairs. The model was initially released only in classic white, but as they continued to grow in popularity they have since been released in many colours, including navy, red and black, and also a model with Velcro straps.

Reissued many times over the years, the rarest and most sought-after shoes are the early models, when Stan's iconic smiling face was stamped in gold. The 'Made in France' issue is also highly sought-after by collectors.

Ignore the posturing of the purists, these are classic shoes that seem to look good with everything. Wear them with pride.

nike
CORTEZ

The Nike Cortez is an obvious entry for the Hall of Fame. Not only is it one of the first shoes ever made by Nike, it also has history with Onitsuka (*see pages 50–1*). More importantly, the shoe is the only model that Nike has continuously produced since its establishment in 1972.

The shoe, now known as the Nike Cortez, had been developed by the forerunner of Nike, Blue Ribbon Sports, in conjunction with the Japanese firm Onitsuka Tiger.

Bill Bowerman, co-founder of Nike, is said to have developed the Cortez by taking apart two pairs of Onitsuka Tigers. He combined the good parts of both, added some ideas of his own, and stitched the result together with an adidas-like 'arch cookie'. The result he sent to Japan and this model eventually became the best-selling Onitsuka Corsair.

After contractual disputes and the subsequent split in dealings with Onitsuka, Nike kept the design, added the now famous 'Swoosh' logo trademark, and renamed the shoe the Nike Cortez. It was launched at the NSGA show in Chicago in February 1972 and went on to become a best-selling model for the company.

The first model was made in leather in the classic colours of white shoe, red Swoosh and a blue line on the side sole. Since the model has spanned such a long production period you can find it in all manner of colours. The shoe was also made in various materials, including nylon and suede, and even the Swoosh changed colour or was sometimes made of imitation crocodile and lizard skin. Colours also varied on the West to East coasts of the United States.

The Cortez became famous as an L.A. gang member's statutory item of footwear, with the Cripps wearing blue or white and the Bloods shod in black. This shoe is still worn around the world by generations who appreciate this design classic.

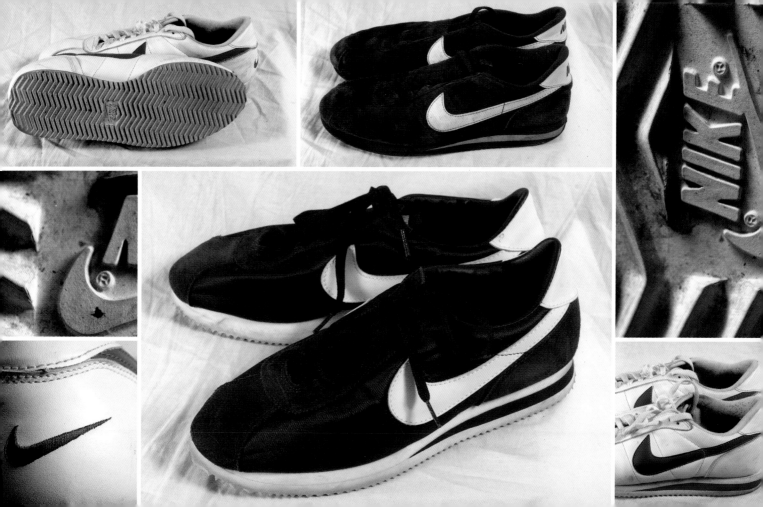

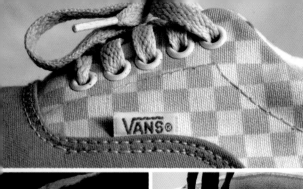
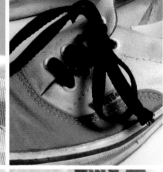
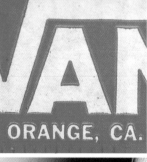
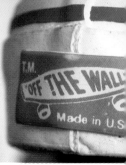
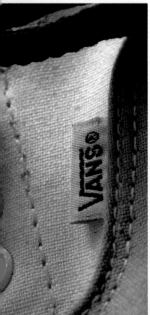
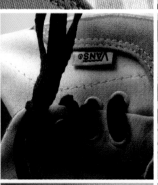
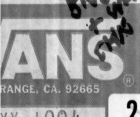
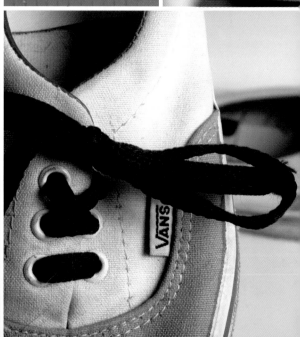
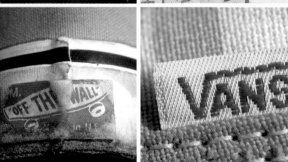

vans

ERA

No matter where you go in the world, there is one sight you are sure to see – urban skater kids dressed in baggy pants, even baggier tops, beanie hats and their all-important footwear. Believe it or not, this 'look' has its origins in a small homegrown youth movement started in southern California in the early 1970s.

It was then that the initial skate kids started to wear the 'deck shoes' that had been developed by a local company with a unique attitude to designing and selling sneakers. That company was Vans, and its story is told later (*see pages 328–9*).

The main reason the early skate gangs, such as now famous Z-Boys, started to wear the initial Vans models, such as the 'Authentic', was that the soles of the shoes were very thick, making them resistant to the punishing treatment of skating. As well, the shoes were cheap and, amazingly, you could even customize them to your own taste. It was possible to 'invent' your own colour combination shoes or, for just $1 extra, use your own material as the upper part of the shoe.

By 1976 the sight of skateboarding kids wearing their customized Vans was so common that the company decided to involve them in the design process of its new shoes. With the help of such Z-Boys as Tony Alva and Stacy Peralta, padded collars and colour combinations, including blue/red and blue/blue, were specified and put into production.

The result was model 95, better known as the Era – the first shoe specifically designed with skateboarding in mind and the first to use the now legendary 'Off the Wall' label on the rear of its heel. The Era has to enter our Hall of Fame, not just because it's a fine looking shoe but also because it was the initiator of a huge industry. The Era, with its padded collar and various colour combinations, became the shoe of choice for an entire generation of skateboarders.

reebok
FREESTYLE

Hindsight is a wonderful thing, but at any particular point in history it is difficult to imagine new developments. In the early 1980s this was the case in the world of trainers. The big players at that time were concentrating their efforts on new shoes for the traditional sporting arena, and this was enough to keep them busy.

However, just when the big boys had taken their eyes off the main prize, a long-established but small-market British player took advantage of the situation. That company was Reebok.

Reebok had roots that went all the way back to 1891, but it wasn't until the late 1970s that the company started to emerge as a global presence in terms of sales. In 1982, it stole a march that pushed it to the top of the trainer sales wars. The product that gave Reebok that competitive edge was the Freestyle.

In the United States, women in particular had been developing a growing passion for fitness, and in the early 1980s a new craze – aerobic dance – was sweeping the country. The demands on footwear now started to shift as these women wanted trainers that were not developed for traditional sports. Aerobics wasn't about sprinting, kicking, or jogging. It involved moving about in a warm gym, or even in your own home in front of a VCR. Aerobic practitioners not only placed a high regard on comfort, but since it was usually a group activity, fashion was important.

Reebok took a keen interest in this fast-growing phenomenon and took the bold step of marketing a trainer specifically designed for women – more particularly, women who practised aerobics – by releasing the shoe in 'female-friendly' pastel shades of hot pink or lemon yellow. The result was spectacular. Within two years a generation of Olivia Newton John-inspired aerobics women propelled Reebok from the minor league to the top of the trainer sales charts.

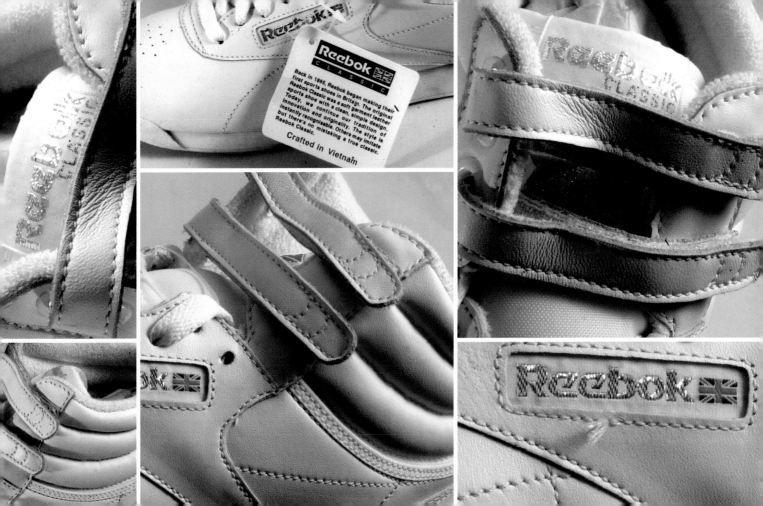

Back in 1895, Reebok began making their first sports shoes in Britain. The original Reebok Classic was a soft garment leather sports shoe with a clean, simple design. Today, we continue our tradition of innovation and originality. The style is instantly recognisable. Others may imitate but there's no mistaking a true classic. Reebok Classic.

Crafted in Vietnam

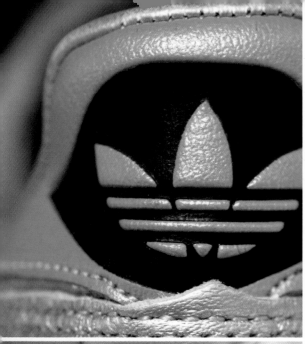

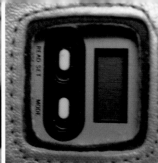

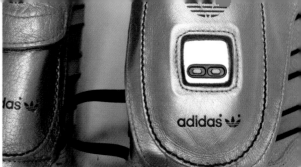

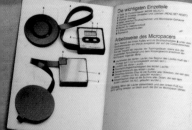

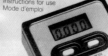

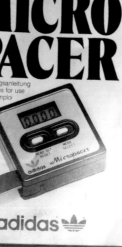

MICRO PACER

Bedienungsanleitung
instructions for use
Mode d'emploi

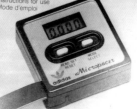

adidas

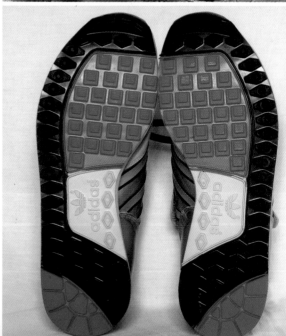

adidas
MICRO PACER

It's 1984 and we have grown used to the sight of trainers as everyday footwear. Obsession has already reared its head. Even so, nothing has prepared us for the latest offering from adidas, the godfather of the brands.

Adidas released the Micro Pacer at a launch tied in with the L.A. Olympics. What hit the stores was so far ahead of its time that its initial failure isn't at all surprising. Aesthetically, the silver leather shoe was shocking. Sneakers simply weren't silver back then. (Actually, the earliest models came in a more mundane light brown colour.) Another first for adidas was the use of colour – a shocking red – in the blocks in the soles. Adidas thought of every detail: on the right foot was a small pocket for your change or keys. However, this shoe's main claim to fame was its innovative on-board technology. The shoe was so advanced that a pair is now displayed in the Computer Museum History Center, in Boston. The technology that caused such a stir was a sensor in the toe connected to a microprocessor embedded in the tongue of the left shoe. The face of the computer resembles a digital LCD watch face. After entering information into the face unit, it calculates the speed, distance and calorific output of the wearer. One drawback, however, is that the clock is only good until the end of 2009.

Like other innovations that are too different for the average buyer, the Micro Pacer was not a big seller initially and was discontinued. The shoe was also expensive (the first to retail at more than $100 in the United States). However, in time, demand grew for this design classic. Adidas reissued it in 2000, with only 600 individually numbered shoes being released on the first run. The demand for the Micro Pacer is still huge, with the sneaker often seen changing hands for considerably more than its original price tag.

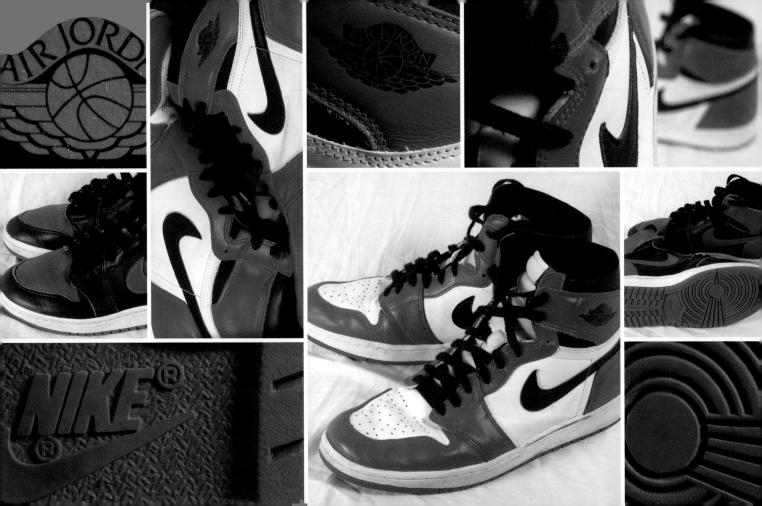

nike
AIR JORDAN 1

Arguably the most famous training shoe in the world was launched in 1985. If Helen of Troy had a face that launched a thousand ships, then the Peter Moore-designed Air Jordan 1 launched a thousand imitations. It is not an overstatement to say that the Air Jordan changed sports for ever.

Whatever you think of the shoe, or the marketing that went with it, there is no denying that the Air Jordan phenomenon practically launched trainers into mass mainstream consciousness on a global scale. More than a million pairs were sold in its first year and it has remained Nike's top-selling basketball shoe ever since. If Air Jordan were a separate sneaker company by itself, then it would be in the top five of industry sales.

Rather aptly, the shoe itself is surrounded by a plethora of urban myths, all helping

to build the legend and to feed the hype. First, the Air Jordan 1 is said to be based on the Giorgio Armani-designed Nike Chicago. Second, and more importantly, the shoe was initially banned by the National Basketball Association (NBA).

At first Michael Jordan wore the black-and-red model because it matched the colours of the Chicago Bulls basketball team. However, the shoe broke league colour rules, which stated that all shoes had to have a white sole base. Marketing-conscious Nike jumped on the free publicity generated and created more hype with its 'Banned by the NBA' commercials, taking the model to the top of the sales charts. After being fined, Jordan mostly wore the white/black-red model instead, and it was in these that he amassed the 'infamous' 63 points score against the Boston Celtics.

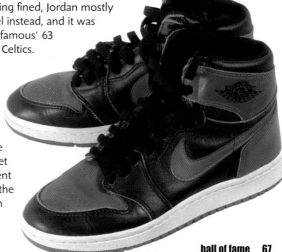

The AJ1 is the only model of the series to feature the Nike Swoosh logo. It is also the model released in the greatest number of colourways (23, to match Jordan's shirt number). The shoes were sold with a double set of laces to match the two different colours, and they are probably the most collectable of all trainers in terms of value.

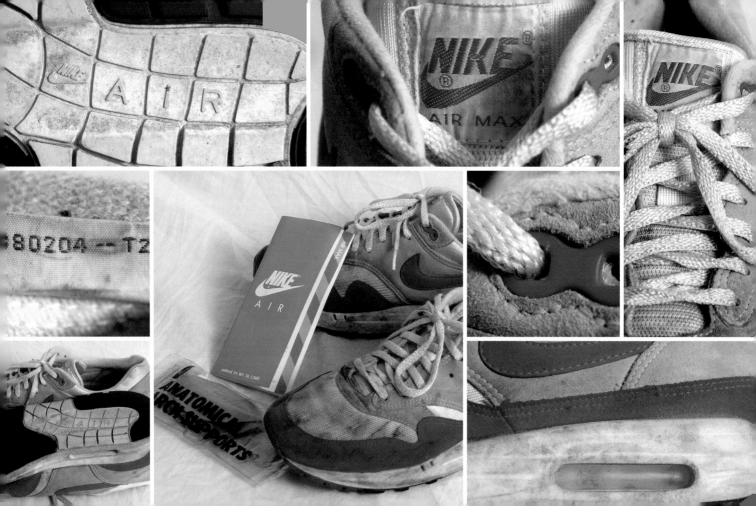

nike
AIR MAX 1

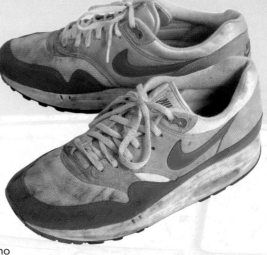

Do we stand still gazing back on the good old days, or do we take our chances and look to the future? When Nike introduced the Air Max 1 in 1987 it certainly was looking to the future. In fact, these shoes were the future. This was the first shoe that aimed to reveal rather than conceal sole technology.

The Air Max 1 was the latest offering in the technological development of the 'Air system'. This system of 'pressurized gas encapsulated in polyurethane' was developed by Marion Frank Rudy, an independent inventor from California who wanted to put small bags of air into shoes to increase performance. Rudy had approached the major training-shoe makers with his idea but it was Nike who recognized its potential. It was one of Phil Knight's better decisions, and one of adidas's worst. Today, framed in the John McEnroe building of the Nike headquarters is the adidas letter of refusal to Frank Rudy for his 'Air system'.

Nike first used the groundbreaking system in 1979 in the Tailwind, the first running shoe with the patented air-sole cushioning system. After further development, the Nike Air 'family' of shoes was introduced with the Air Force 1 and Air Ace in 1982. However, as good as these developments are, it is the Nike Air Max 1 that enters our Hall of Fame, because the simple idea of 'Visible Air' brought this technology to a wider audience.

Basically, the Nike Air Max was the first shoe to let you see its technology within your shoe. Via the use of 'windows' at the front and rear of the shoes, the Air Max allowed you to think that you were at the cutting edge of trainer technology, and bouncing along on air. These special windows also transferred air outside the unit on impact, and this was the development known as 'Maximum Volume'.

Apart from all the technology inside, the shoe was aesthetically head-turning. It is possible to wear the first issue in its classic red/grey/white livery and still look as cool as they come.

reebok

CLASSIC LEATHER

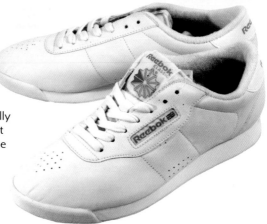

Being just one of the Reebok 'Classic' range of trainers, the Reebok Classic (officially named the Classic Leather) was released in 1987, but it is such a familiar shoe that it seems to have been around for much longer. The model has now appropriated the 'Classic' name, and when anybody speaks of Reebok Classics, or even 'Classics', only one shoe springs to mind. As another of the 'cultural' entrants into the Hall of Fame, no list of trainers would be complete without it.

The Classic (to use its common name) is the biggest-selling single model of trainer in the U.K. today. It is seen everywhere, every day and on every street corner. Strangely, the shoe seems to have no cultural boundaries and easily crosses over the different genres of inner-city youth culture, and is seen most often in its purest white 'Bling Bling' form. The popularity of the Classics among the older generation also cannot be underestimated. And due to the comfort factor, the Classic is also popular with supermarket-visiting mothers.

Even though the initial beginnings of this shoe are clouded in urban folklore, this particular piece of folklore happens to be true. When Reebok was developing the model for production, there was a misorder at the factory, which resulted in the delivery of some hyper-supple kangaroo leather. With time at a premium, the shoes were made up using the now famous kangaroo hide and a 'Classic' shoe came into being. It was the very nature of this 'mistake' that gave rise to the shoe's popularity. Love it or hate it, there is no denying that this trainer is incredibly comfortable to wear.

And the particular look and feel that came about as a result has given it a unique aesthetic.

However, for a shoe that is so universally popular, it sure takes a lot of stick. Curiously, even though it is so popular, and even though Reebok is the only British brand to be part of the 'big few', it is adidas that has brand loyalty among the British trainer purists, with Reebok receiving more respect 'across the pond' in the United States.

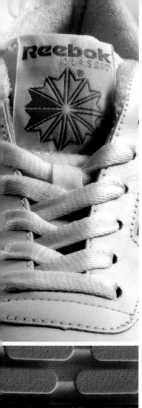
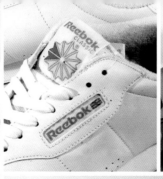
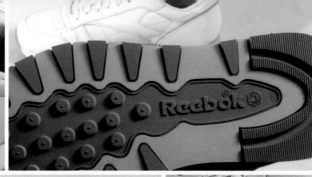
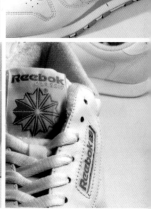
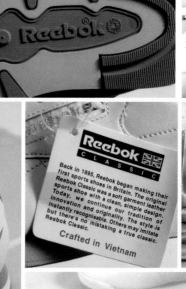

Back in 1895, Reebok began making their first sports shoes in Britain. The original Reebok Classic was a soft garment leather sports shoe with a clean, simple design. Today, we continue our tradition of innovation and originality. The style is instantly recognisable. Others may imitate but there's no mistaking a true classic. Reebok Classic.

Crafted in Vietnam

Shoe Care Instructions

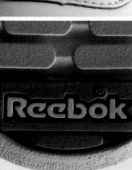
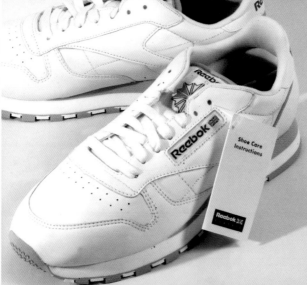
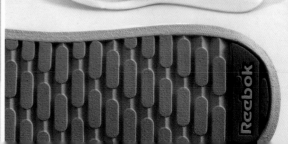

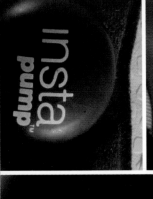

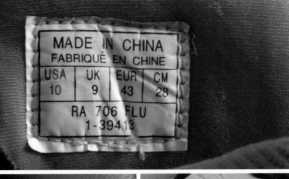

MADE IN CHINA
FABRIQUÉ EN CHINE

USA	UK	EUR	CM
10	9	43	28

RA 706 FLU
1-39418

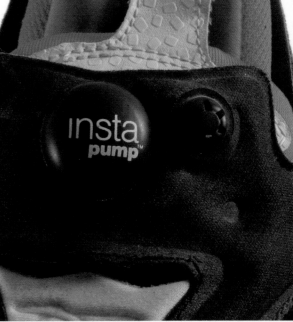

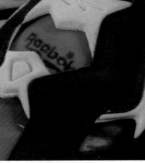

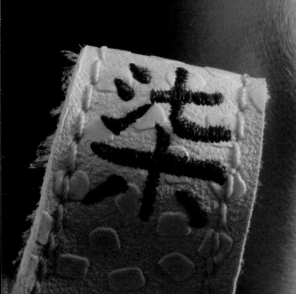

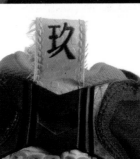

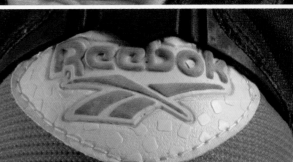

reebok
INSTAPUMP

Every design process seems to have a 'Holy Grail' among the design community. For trainers, this seemed to be the humble lace. For some reason, something that had been around for years as a perfectly practical and aesthetic detail was there to be shot at by the trainer firms. Call it a gimmick or just plain tinkering, the 'laceless shoe' had been a goal for some time. Nike had approached the idea of using air to aid fit with its Nike Air Pressure model. Reebok went one step further, and better, with the introduction of the Reebok Pump in 1989. But, it was the introduction of the Reebok Instapump Fury in 1994 that finally saw the dream fulfilled. The laceless trainer.

To add to the shock of the new, the designers at Reebok who worked on the shoe, such as Paul Litchfield and Steven Smith, decided they should give the shoe even more impact by producing it in 'crazy' neon colours. The shoe's first release was in neon yellow, red and black.

The whole aim of the shoe was to customize fit without using laces. But it wasn't just this that made the design stand out. Yes, Reebok had achieved the laceless trainer but they had also dramatically altered the look. Gone was the full-length sole seen in every other shoe to date. Instead there was a big 'gap' in the middle of the sole unit (officially named 'full-foot low-chamber technology') as well as a hole in the side of the shoe. The Fury also used stretch material containing a pumpable bladder system in order to gain a snug fit.

Basically once slipped on the foot, you could engage the shoe's simple pump system by depressing the main 'pumping unit button' on the 'tongue'. By pressing this rubber button it was possible to inflate a built-in inflatable tongue, or bladder, to provide a secure and comfortable fit. For once, a design gimmick actually worked.

Again, like the few trainers that are truly groundbreaking, the Instapump elicits strong emotions – you either love it or you hate it. Whatever camp you are in, it deserves a place in this Hall of Fame for its innovative design concept.

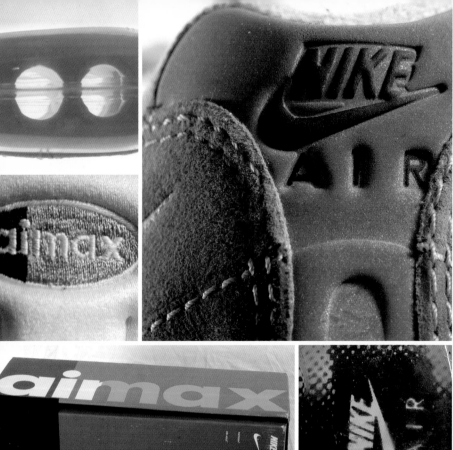

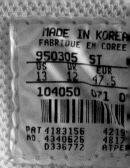
13
UK 12
EUR 47.5
CM 31

AIR MAX

BLACK/NEON YEL
MADE IN KOREA
FABRIQUE EN CO

104050

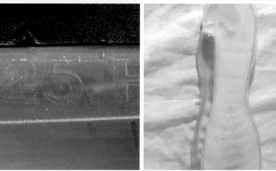

MADE IN KOREA
FABRIQUE EN COREE
950305 ST
US UK EUR
13 12 47.5
104050 D71 0
PAT 4183156 4219
NO. 4340625 4817
D336772 ATPE

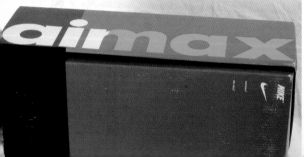

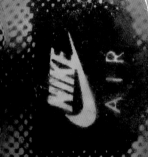

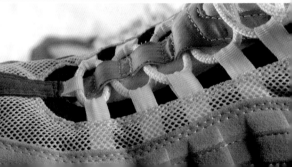

nike
AIR MAX 95

Back in 1995 when I first saw these shoes, I actually thought they were plain ugly, but so utterly mad that I had to buy them... and then I didn't take them off for a whole year! This shoe was the Air Max 95.

Officially, the shoe is called the Air Total Max, because its designer, Serfio Lorenzo, wanted to express his desire for something 'total', the best. It's debatable whether he ever achieved this aim, but he certainly changed the course of trainer development. For good or for bad, this was the first shoe to make mainstream fashion houses sit up and take notice of trainer design.

The Air Max 95 was the first model in which Nike adopted the 'visible air' unit at the front of the shoe. Before this, shoes such as the Nike Tailwind had used total air cushioning, and since 1987 there had been the visible rear air unit of the Air Max 1.

But it wasn't any small technical change that made such a mark on trainer evolution – it was the total package. The shoe was just different, like something discarded by fleeing aliens. It had a particularly high-tech look, the colours were different (acid yellow and green), there was a reflective panel, and the whole shoe was covered in strange contours. And to add to the impact, he used those neon colours against shades of grey and black.

Also, the mesh gave it even more of an alien feel, which added to the focus on the technical detailing of the air bubbles. Not only that, the air bubbles were huge and

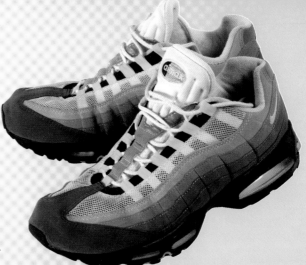

everywhere. The one understated part of the whole design was the Swoosh, which was tucked away at the rear of the shoe.

Lorenzo had actually been inspired by the human body: the clear part on the sole mimics the backbone, the graduation of the upper represents the muscles and the bumpy part the ribs. Either love it or loathe it, this shoe can't be ignored and rightly takes its place in the Hall of Fame.

nike
AIR WOVEN

It was the year 2000, the dawn of the new millennium, and the Nike Air Woven was released upon an unsuspecting world. What better date to start a revolution? The Woven is the most recently issued shoe in our Hall of Fame, and is also probably the most controversial entry.

The shoe, designed by Mike Aveni at Nike, was produced by allying a woven interlocked, elasticated construction to a running-shoe air sole. The result is similar to the sort of summer loafers warn by the smartly dressed, but it also tugs at a more rural tradition reminiscent of basket weaving, or something you cannot quite put your finger on. Despite this it still looks totally new and modern.

The Air Woven was first released in Tokyo (a demanding arena full of trainer addicts),

before going on to London and New York. The hype surrounding the shoe was surprisingly low-key, and this helped to fuel demand when it was released. No one really had any idea it was coming.

In every country of issue, public response on its initial release was universally the same: the term 'mad' or 'crazy' had probably never been applied so frequently and in so many different languages to a shoe. The Woven was probably also the shoe most likely never to be worn by its first owner. It sparked a mini economic boom in trainer trade as 'sneaker speculators' around the globe bought the shoes and immediately put them on sale to a Woven-hungry public. The boom in sales was partly a result of the Woven having been released in a different colour for each country. At the height of the craze, shoes were often seen changing hands at a minimum of 50 per cent more than their initial cost.

However, the debate is not about cost or personal taste, but more about breaking new ground. The shoe made us think about what direction trainers could take or, more to the point, what direction was out of bounds. Anything now seemed possible.

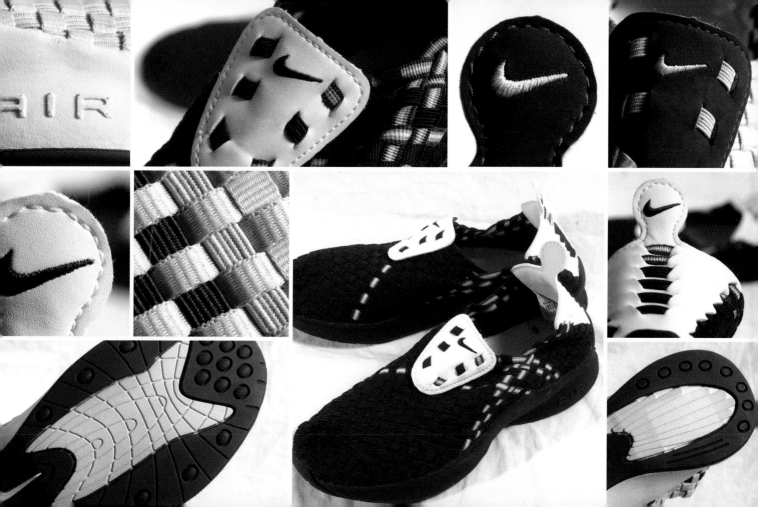

trainers & popular culture

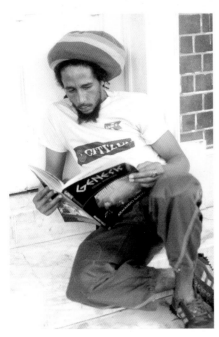

You know you've got it bad when all you can do when watching films or old classic cop shows from the 1970s is look for the trainers the stars are wearing. I knew I had it bad when watching war scenes in Afghanistan – I found myself looking to see which old adidas classics the Mujahadin were wearing.

Many musicians have written about their shoes. Run DMC had *Me and my adidas*, while up and coming British band The Streets have recently sung about their Reebok Classics. It does not stop there – Bob Marley was so into adidas that he had his own strips made for himself and the band. Converse shoes have featured

in over 150 films and there are websites detailing where you can Chuck Taylor spot. It didn't take long for the brands to take notice and develop product placement in a big way. Of course, marketing-aware Nike were there first. It is a Nike co-developed shoe that Marty Mcfly sports in *Back to the Future* (part II).

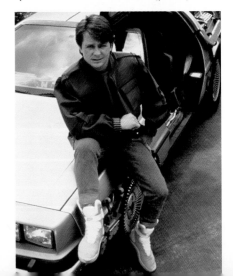

LEFT Adidas fan Bob Marley relaxes in his TRX.
RIGHT Marty McFly (Michael J. Fox) in custom-made Nikes developed from the Air Pressure model.

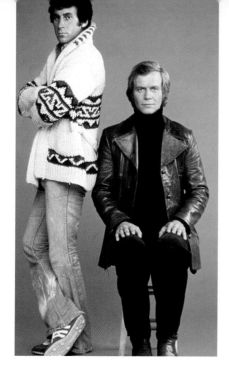

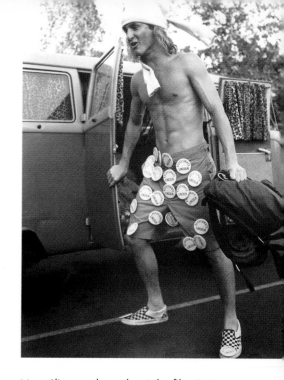

LEFT Icons of the 1970s, super-cops Starsky and Hutch could often be seen wearing adidas trainers.
RIGHT Sean Penn popularizing Vans sneakers on the big screen.

Here we detail just a few of the famous trainer-inspired film scenes and bands. So go on, get out there and search for examples yourself, too.

STARSKY AND HUTCH
Like a lot of films and programmes from the 1970s, Starsky and Hutch is great for trainer spotting. Usually the boys would be seen posing about town in adidas Dragons, among others.

FAST TIMES AT RIDGEMONT HIGH
Sean Penn was one of the original skaters and would bus down from Malibu to hit the streets with Tony Alva and the Z-Boys. Vans were amazingly popular with the skate kids, but when Penn was seen in his chequerboard

Who do you think organized the *Forest Gump* scene when Tom Hanks lifts a pair of Nike Cortez from the box for the world to see? Anyway, the list goes on and on, and once you start looking, you can't stop.

Vans Slip-ons throughout the film *Fast Times at Ridgemont High* the shoes really took off. One famous scene had Penn hitting himself about the head with these classic Vans.

GAME OF DEATH

Bruce Lee gets in on the act in many martial arts films and, keeping the Asian flavour, he can be seen in an early pair of Onitsuka Tigers, ready to kung-fu kick someone into hyperspace with the Japanese trainers on his feet.

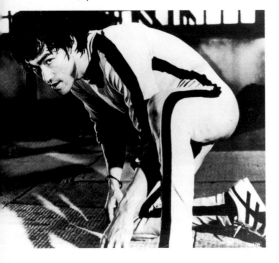

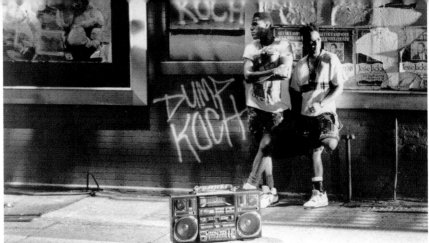

ABOVE From *Do the Right Thing*.
LEFT Bruce Lee in Onitsuka Tigers.

DO THE RIGHT THING

This film was almost an extended Nike sneaker advertisement. Made in 1989, the film-maker Spike Lee became heavily involved with future Nike promotions. The film features up to 80 per cent of the characters wearing Nikes, but one particularly famous scene sees a pair of precious Jordan 4s being run over by a car.

OTHER FAMOUS FILMS

• In the cult-classic *Terminator*, watch Arnie blow people away in his now overtly popular Vandals.
• Nike Dunk-clad Jack Nicholson in *The Witches of Eastwick* plays the quintessential bad boy.
• Sly Stallone's Rocky changes allegiance throughout his films. In *Rocky 1*, he is always wearing Converse, but by *Rocky 3* he has become a Nike man. However, in *Rocky 4* he is sporting adidas, while his cornerman wears Diadora.

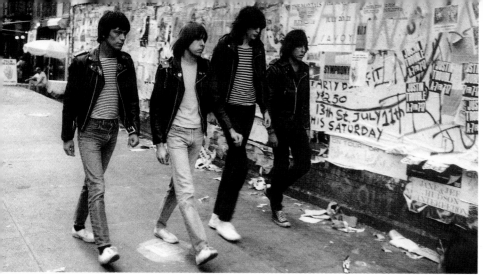

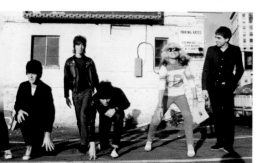

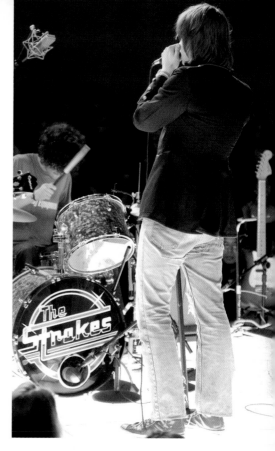

ABOVE New York band The Ramones wearing Hi and Lo Kicks.
LEFT Debbie Harry (in heels), with the rest of Blondie in their 'Canvas' sneakers. Blondie members show the trainer tradition that is taken on today by The Strokes in their adherence to canvas basket shoes, particularly Converse Chucks or Keds and Sperries.
RIGHT The Strokes in Chucks.

sporting connections

Interestingly, when you stop to look at it, the field of sporting endorsements is not the modern phenomenon that we sometimes imagine and, depressingly, the curse of celebrity obsession is not something that the present generation has sole rights to. This effect of celebrity endorsement has had a significant impact in the world of trainers. In fact, it could be said that the trainer world was at it before anybody else.

If you look at the shoes that are either among the best-selling models of all time or are of great repute, then you can almost guarantee that a great proportion of the them will be 'signature shoes'. That is, shoes with the endorsement of a sporting celebrity.

Indeed, one of the first 'official' trainers of all time is a case in point when, during 1916, Converse released the humble All Star basketball shoe. However, it was in 1923, when ex-basketball player Chuck Taylor had his name added to the trainer – thus creating the first sporting 'signature shoe' – that the shoe really took off with the buying public.

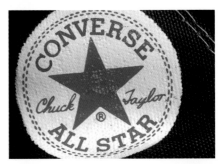

The adidas Stan Smith started life as the adidas Robet Haillet in 1956. But it was in 1971 when, in an early instance of 'celebrity fit', the now famous smiling face was added to the tongue. The smiling face that greets every wearer is that of American tennis player Stan Smith. It was only when he added his endorsement to the shoe that it achieved greater public awareness and went on to become the classic it is today.

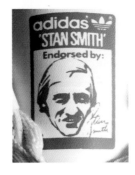
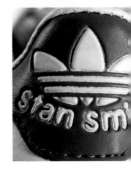

TOP RIGHT Converse displaying the first endorsee, Chuck Taylor.
RIGHT Adidas and Stan Smith, loud and proud.

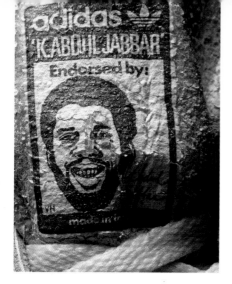

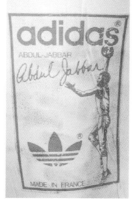

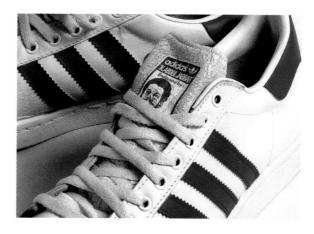

FAR RIGHT The Jabbar was created for NBA star Kareem Abdul Jabbar.
MIDDLE The original Jabbar tongue with the Sky Hook.
ABOVE Jabbar's smiling face.

The Puma State or Suede, as the trainer is variously known, was a popular shoe right from its initial launch in 1968. However, it was not until 1974, when the then famous basketball player Walt Clyde

Frazier added his name to the model, thus creating the Clyde, that sales really took off for the company.

Another notable endorsement was secured by adidas when it included the happy face of Kareem Abdul Jabbar, an early 1970s' basketball player, on the the tongue of its trainer. Other notable 'faces' shoes spawned by adidas include tennis superstars Illie Nastase and Billie Jean King.

Puma carried off another of their significant coups in the soccer field when it captured the endorsement of the great Pele. The Brazilian worked closely with Puma on the model's development and his range of shoes went on to do very well for the German brand.

However, the field of sporting endorsements at that time was not as we know it today. Then, endorsees might

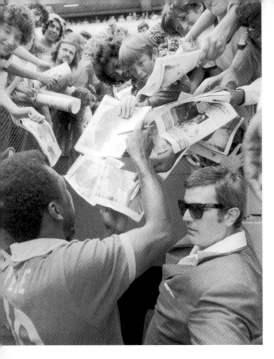

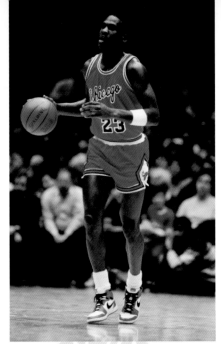

their sales. Undoubtedly the most famous and most successful endorsement of all time can be explained in two words: Air Jordan.

LEFT Puma endorsee and probably the world's most famous soccer player, Pelé, being mobbed by autograph-hunting fans.

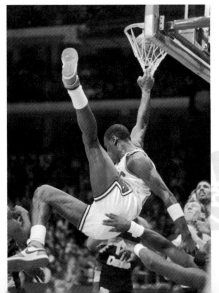

wear one Reebok and one Diadora shoe at the same time in order to keep both sponsors happy. It really took the introduction of one particular Nike model and its celebrity endorsement to change the whole profile of training shoes and

ABOVE The man himself, Michael Jordan wearing a pair of his own endorsed shoes, the AJ 1.
LEFT Nike's top-selling basketball shoes ever – Jordan 1s in action doing what made them famous.

Michael Jordan was an up-and-coming basketball rookie who wore only adidas or Converse, but it was Nike that made one of its best moves when it persuaded him to add his name to its shoes in 1985. The success of the Jordan series has been unparalleled and the basketball star has the final say on the design of the shoes bearing his name each year.

Endorsements were not always sporting in nature and in the crazy 1980s Michael Jackson designed a total new range for L.A. Gear, including the Billie Jeans complete with studs, leather and buckles to match his video.

RIGHT TOP Tennis superstar, Andre Agassi, in Nike Air Tech Challenge, commonly known as 'Agassis'.
RIGHT BOTTOM LEFT Boxer Frank Bruno giving his all for Nike.
FAR RIGHT Soccer player George Best gets in on the act and adds his name to a pair of trainers.

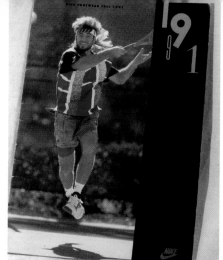

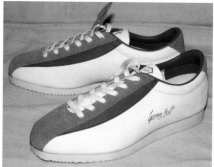

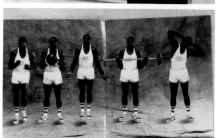

ANYTHING HE WANTS.

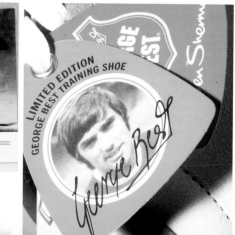

LIMITED EDITION
GEORGE BEST TRAINING SHOE

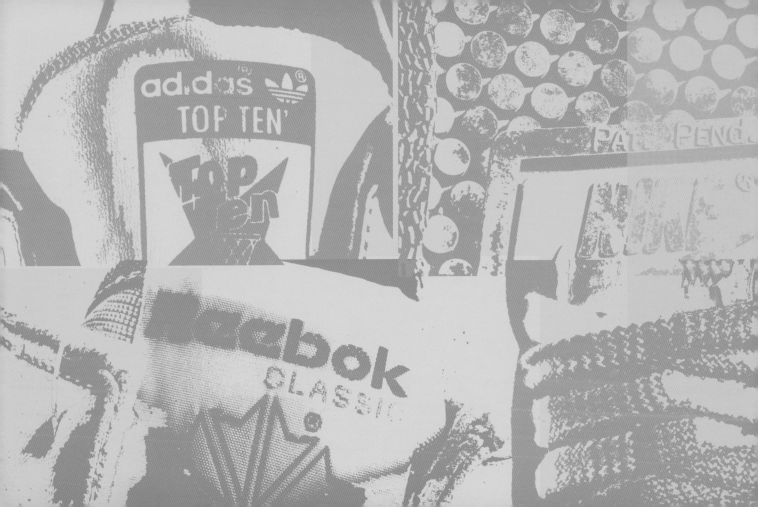

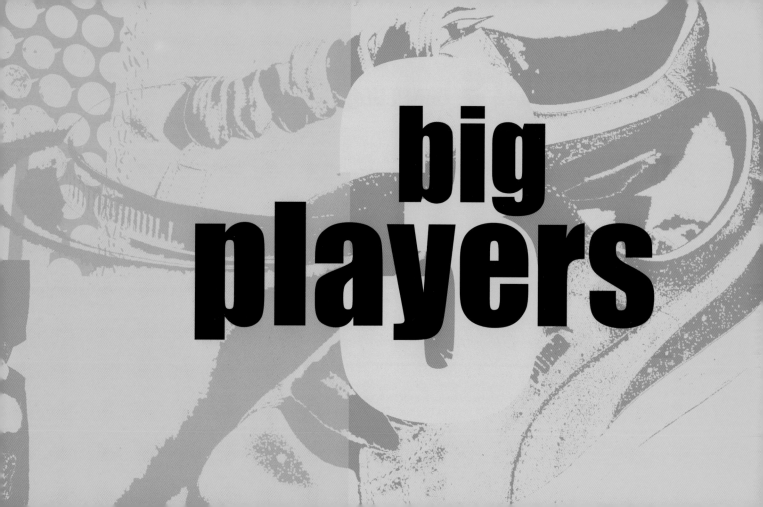

big
players

big players every dog has its day

INTRODUCTION

Although a lot of attention is paid to market performance and to market share, sales alone do not guarantee entry into the annals of trainer respect.

As in most fields of commercial activity, the training shoe brands experience their fair share of ups and downs. And as reputations go in and out of fashion, so market share moves substantially from decade to decade – indeed, even from month to month.

In addition, brand 'presence' varies significantly from country to country, and while a particular brand might be selling well in one market it could well be simultaneously falling in another. If, for example, you asked a couple of kids who they thought were big players in the trainer world, the answers would depend on where you asked the question.

At the moment, no matter where you are in the world, you would probably hear the name Nike mentioned in reply. However, this has not always been the case and will probably not always be so in the future.

In the 1960s and up until the early 1970s the brands that could claim to be 'big players' would certainly have been the giant German companies adidas and Puma. The only other competitors worth mentioning then were Converse in America, Dunlop and Gola in the U.K., and Onitsuka in Japan. Other countries had many and varied sports-shoe producers: Finland has to this day Karhu, with its brilliant Bear logo; Italy had Diadora and Bata, with Fila adding in later to the mix. The list could go on and on. However, the point really is that, rather like boy bands today, trainer

brands may be extremely well known in one particular country while being virtually unknown just across the border.

By the mid 1970s this situation had began to change. Onitsuka sneakers, under the guidance of Blue Ribbon Sports (the early incarnation of Nike), were imported into the United States to break the dominance of the Germans. Nike itself was launched only as recently as 1972, and took until the mid-1980s to become the main player that it is today. In 1977 Reebok hit the States and rapidly developed into the major force it now is.

The 1980s was the decade of the 'Trainer Wars'. This was when the training-shoe phenomenon really took off and brand awareness and sales became a huge business. Advertising also played a major part as trainers made the move from the

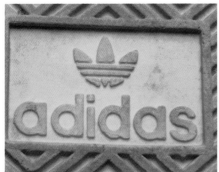

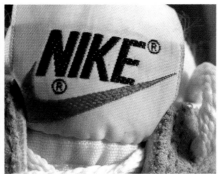

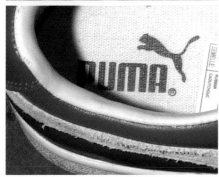

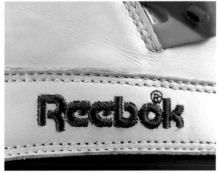

sporting field to become the basic leisurewear item that we now recognize.

This leads us back to the opening statement opposite: 'every dog has its day'. During the 1980s, all sorts of odd brands gained market share almost overnight. Brands such as L.A. Gear, British Knights and Brooks jumped into the market in order to snap up a piece of the burgeoning leisurewear and fashion market. L.A. Gear went from second spot in terms of sales to a market share of just 1 per cent in less than a decade.

Therefore, when drawing up our list of big players, both longevity and sporting development were major considerations. Hence, we arrive at a list containing adidas, Nike, Puma and Reebok. This is not to say that others, such as Converse or Dunlop, haven't played their part, but the big players have been at the top for some time and have been significantly involved in the sporting field.

adidas brand history

Our story begins in the town of Herzogenaurach, near Nuremberg, Germany. As small as it is, this town has had a huge impact on the story of the training shoe. Part of the significant role played by Herzogenaurach takes place in 1948, for this is the year that the aptly nicknamed 'Godfather' of training shoes, adidas, is launched on the world.

A cobbler working in Herzogenaurach, Adolph Dassler, decides on a name for his new company. By combining his nickname 'Adi' with the first three letters of his surname Dassler, the name 'adidas' is born. Apparently Dassler decided to use a lowercase 'a' for the company name to further distinguish it from the competition. By the time of his death in 1978, at the age of 78, Adi Dassler held more than 700 patents related to sports shoes and other athletic equipment, and had also gaining the honour of becoming the first non-American to be inducted into the American Sporting Goods Industry Hall of Fame. Adidas was also a groundbreaking company away from the sports field and was the first sports brand to sponsor non-athletes (Run DMC).

THE DASSLER BROTHERS

Even though adidas came into being in 1948, its history goes back to 1920. A story well known in trainer circles that is worth repeating here concerns the fact that the history of adidas and Puma are intertwined. Thus, to look at the beginnings of adidas you also have to look at the beginnings of Puma.

The story of both adidas and Puma starts back in Herzogenaurach, where Adi's father, who was also a cobbler, and brother Rudolph ('Rudi') lived. Both the boys, Adi and

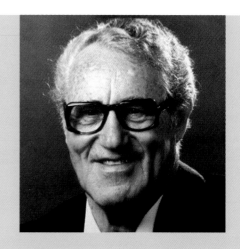

ABOVE The man himself, adidas founder Adolph (Adi) Dassler.

Rudi, were keen sports enthusiasts but, the story goes, Adi was never satisfied with the fit of his sports shoes. So, being the son of a cobbler, he started to make his own. The shoes began to gain a reputation and as the orders came in and the business grew, the brothers decided

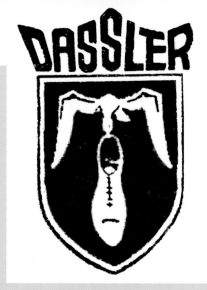

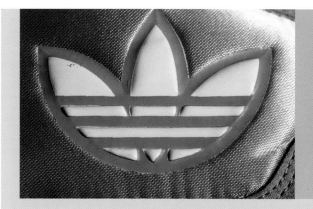

LEFT The well-known trefoil (sometimes called clover) logo used by adidas is said to have come from the motif of the laurel crown given to the winners of sporting festivals in ancient Greece. The crown represented the Olympic spirit and the pursuit of victory.

ABOVE The original Dassler logo used before the family split.

to form a company, which they registered as Gebrüder Dassler OHG (Dassler Brothers Ltd) on 1 July 1924.

The company's success continued, and the Dassler brothers supplied shoes for the German teams at both the 1928 and 1932

Olympics, with models such as the Waitzer and Dassler. However, one notable historic moment for the Dassler brothers came when the prominent black American athlete Jesse Owens won four gold medals at the 1936 Berlin Olympics in front of a furious Adolph Hitler. And the shoes Owens wore for these famous historic victories? Why, Dasslers, of course.

The biggest change in the fortunes of the two brothers was still to come. In 1948, a dispute broke out between Adi and Rudi. Rumours for the split abounded, the usual suspects being women and money. Whatever the real reasons, the rift proved impossible to heal and they finally decided to go their own ways. Adolph left and formed adidas while Rudi moved across town to start Puma. After a few years of legal disputes, each company developed into a worldwide brand in its own right.

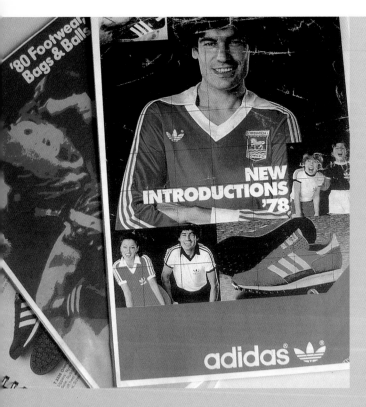

In 1949 adidas added the now legendary three stripes to its trainers as a means of strengthening the shoe and providing extra stability to the foot, and a world-recognized trademark was launched.

In 1966 the first rights to distribute adidas in the United States were taken by H.B. 'Doc' Hughes of Dallas, and the brand quickly became responsible for the biggest-selling training shoes in the country. The 1960s and 70s can rightly be described as being dominated by adidas and Puma, and in 1971 yet another event of huge sporting magnitude took place – Muhammad Ali and Joe Frazier both wore adidas boxing shoes in their 'fight of the century'. In 1972, in the same year that adidas was named official supplier for the Munich Olympics, adidas introduced one of the most recognizable and much loved logos in the world – the adidas 'trefoil'.

Throughout that decade the adidas brand stayed strong, despite increased competition, especially that from an upstart company in business only since 1972 – Nike. After Adi's death in 1978 the running of adidas passed to family members, but by 1987 the company had fallen into the hands of an outsider.

At the start of the 1990s adidas was on the slide from its once dominant position, and the company passed to the since disgraced

LEFT Catalogues and advertisements from the 1970s and 1980s.

Bernard Taupie, the man who had tried to buy the outcome of soccer's prestigious European Cup Final in favour of his own Olympique Marseilles F.C.

In 1996, in an attempt to rebrand and rebuild sales, a new logo was introduced, replacing the classic trefoil with the now familiar three stripes.

Since then, adidas stock has been moved about between various owners, and what started out as a German family business is now a unit of a French global concern – Solomon. Unfortunately, due to what appears to be a lack of focus in brand identity, adidas lost its way and was in urgent need of redefining.

However, throughout the history of trainer companies, market domination comes and goes. In the mid 1970s the top eight trainer companies were characterized as 'adidas and the Seven Dwarves'. And even though adidas may not currently be the major player in the worldwide trainer marketplace, you need to bear the old saying 'form is temporary, class is permanent' firmly in mind.

Even though Converse, Dunlop and Keds were all producing sporting shoes in one form or another first, it is adidas that can rightly lay claim to being the godfather of the trainer brands.

RIGHT The 'performance' adidas logo has been in use since late 1991. It started out specifically for the Equipment range and is probably not as widely recognized nor as fondly thought of as the original trefoil logo, which is synonymous with the brand.

ADIDAS AND THE U.K.

In the long and often ill-tempered history of Anglo-German relationships over the centuries, there is one curious anomaly – the love and loyalty that the youth of the U.K. have reserved for their adidas trainers. Such is the degree of affection for these shoes that it is sometimes surprisingly easy to forget that adidas is not actually a British company.

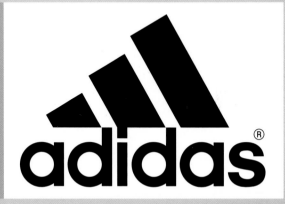

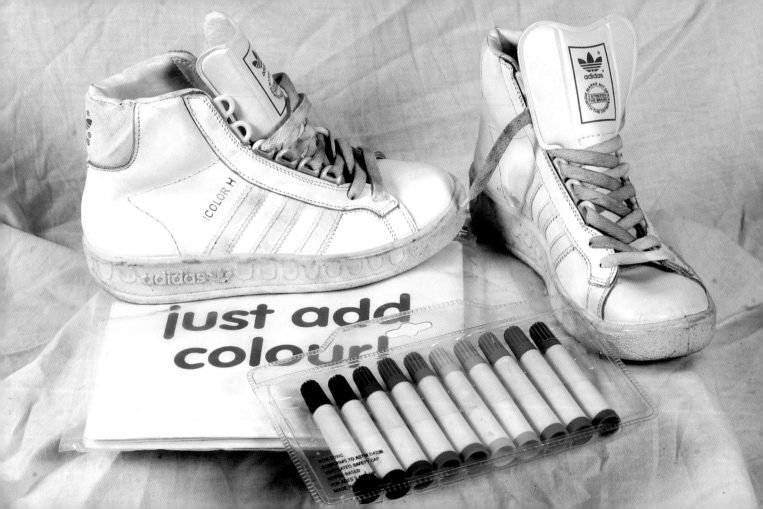

adi colour

For a brand known primarily for sporting initiatives, adidas sure took risks at times, and Adi Colour was a case in point. Released as an interactive shoe, it came in plain white, with its three stripes to match. Adidas also supplied a set of indelible marker pens so that you could colour the shoe as you thought best. The shoes came in both hi and lo versions.

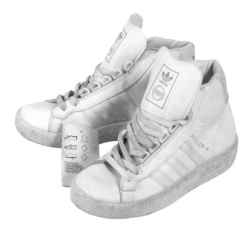

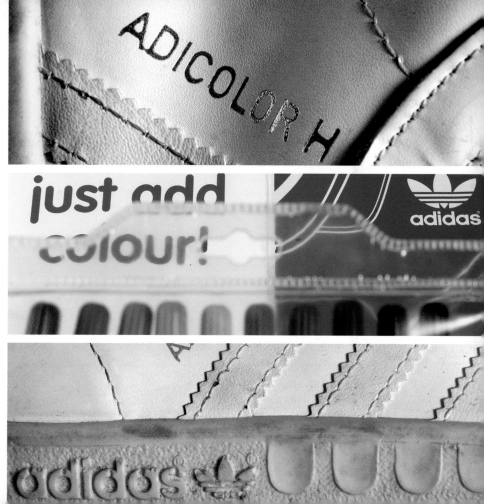

all black

One of the 'Black shoe series' of trainers from adidas is the All Black. Sharing 'stable room' with the Sambas, Kicks and Bambas of the same era, this sneaker was produced in 1981 and the model was designed initally as an indoor soccer perfomance shoe. Now, the All Black is a very rare item indeed.

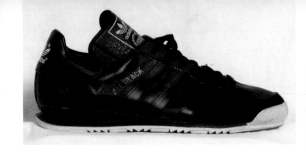

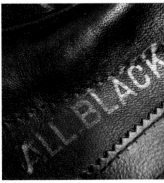

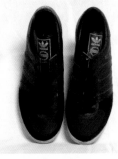

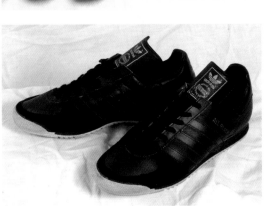

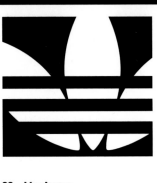

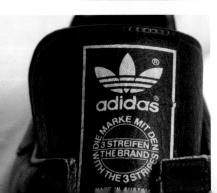

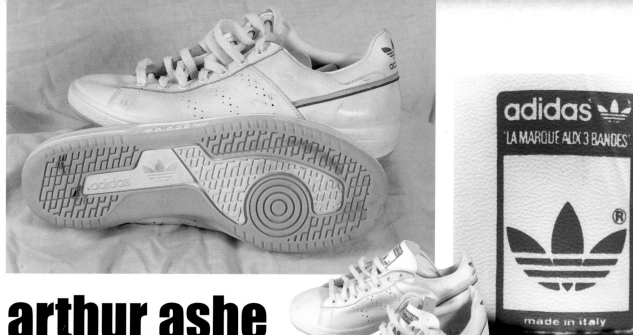

arthur ashe

This is the rarest of the sporting-endorsed adidas tennis series, bearing the name of the first black tennis champion. Resembling the Stan Smith with leather uppers, the model also featured the same perforation holes, which replaced the three stripes. The shoe came in white with red at the heel and, rarely for adidas, the name is also on the heel.

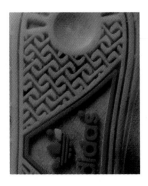
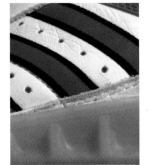
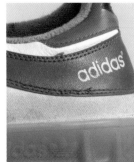

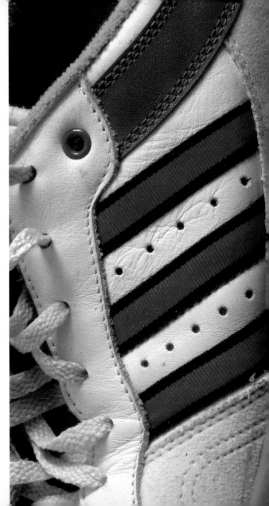

No prizes for guessing which sport these trainers were designed for. This top-of-the-range badminton shoe was produced in the early 1980s and it managed to shed something of the 'flimsy' look of earlier indoor-racket sports shoes. The extra cash also bought you longer-lasting leather as well as other higher specifications.

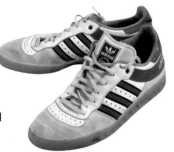

badminton super

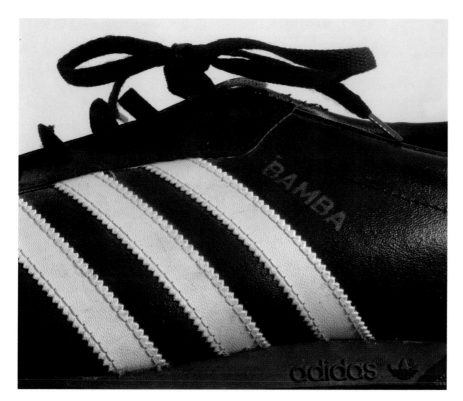

bamba

This early adidas model was released as a football shoe, designed especially for icy or frozen ground. The Bamba is the baby brother of the classic and more expensive Samba and, being only partly made of leather, it was a cheaper option. One of the Black series of adidas models, it was not available in any other colour (apart from its three white stripes).

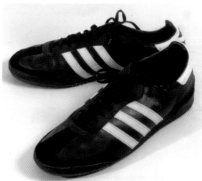

barcelona

This shoe takes its place with the other famous European 'City' series, such as the London and Dublin, produced by adidas, and it is one of the few of this kind we have detailed in the book. The Barcelona is a later additions to the series and sports the same silhouette and chunky polyurethane sole unit as the Trimm Trab.

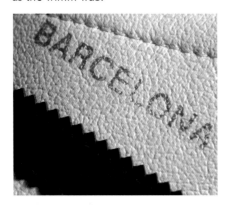

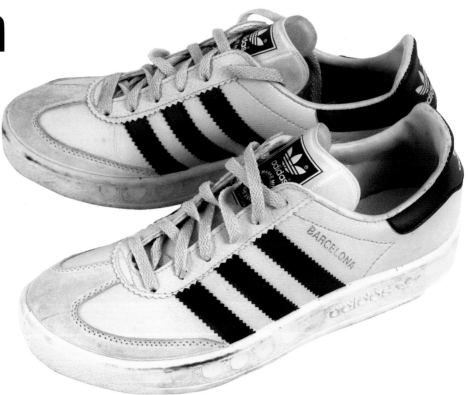

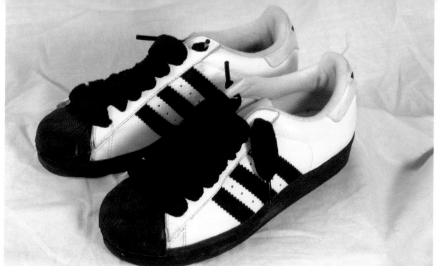

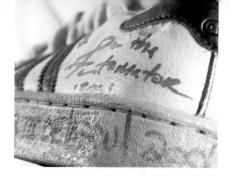

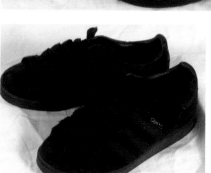

campus

The **Campus** is another from the adidas stable that seems constantly to be on release and popular. The shoe was first issued in the early 1970s and has sold well ever since. Most famously known for its leather version with the 'superstar' shell toe, the model is just as regularly seen without this feature. The sneaker was also released in a suede version without the shell. It was initially available in sky blue, navy and burgundy.

centaur

This early 1980s' running shoe was popular with the Casuals (*see pages 14–9*) and was one of the precursors of the later ZX series that was developed by adidas. The shoes employed early advances in technology; the two-colourway sole units are shared by the Micro Pacer, among others, and are designed to increase stability and flexibility.

concord

A classic basketball shoe from adidas and another example of a shoe on the cutting edge of design, materials and imagination. This example, in fake snakeskin, would be considered mad if released today, never mind the early 1980s. The original came in a shiny blue enamel finish. The ankle strap added stability and was an aesthetically superb feature.

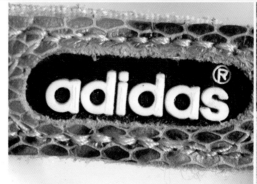
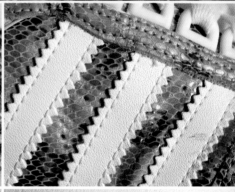
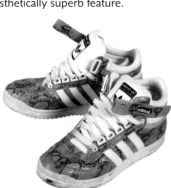
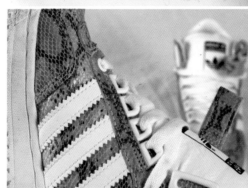
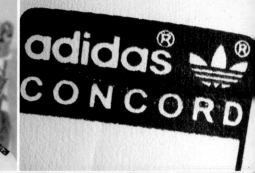

country

This original adidas running silhouette was first launched in 1970 as a cross-country shoe, but is now more likely to be seen on feet in any city across the globe. It is one of the adidas range that consistently sells as a 'classic'. The shoe is made of full-grain leather with a rubber herringbone outsole. The shoe was sold under the slogan: 'Run longer. Run faster. Run smarter.'

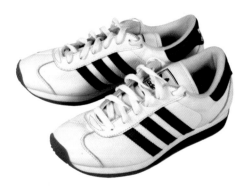

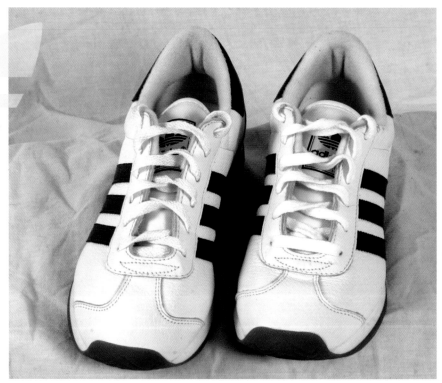

dublin

Developed by adidas in the late 1970s/early 1980s as one of the 'City' series of shoes, the Dublin is included in this book as part of the 'Leisure' category. The City models are interesting as they were a notable step away from performance shoes. With the leisure market particularly in mind, the colours adidas employed were extremely important, and this Dublin model exhibits the same silhouette, flat sole and coloured suede upper design common to the 'European Capital City' series. These sneakers were popular with the soccer-following public, too.

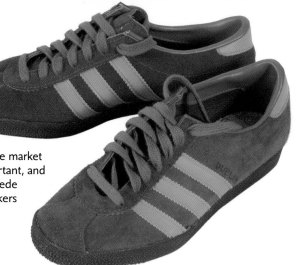

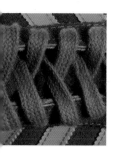
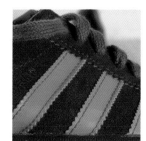
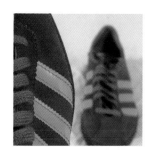
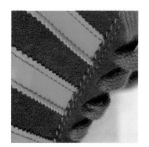
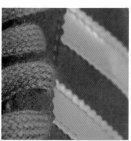
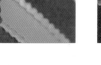

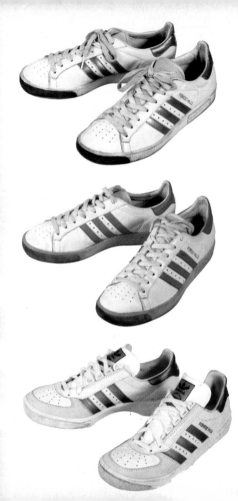

forest hills

Released in the late 1970s as a tennis shoe, the Forest Hills has gained legendary status, particularly with U.K. soccer fans. One of the myths surrounding it was that many people claimed to have owned the yellow-soled version when it was reissued. However, only 400 pairs of them originally entered the U.K. – and they were all bought by Wade Smith in Liverpool. The ordinary shoe had a white sole.

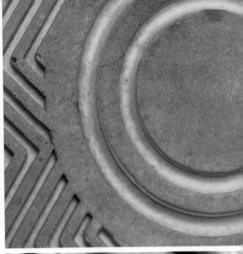

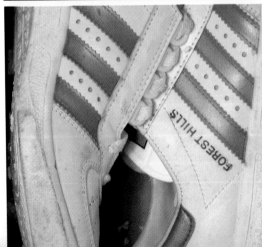

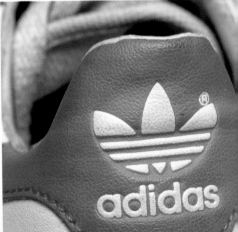

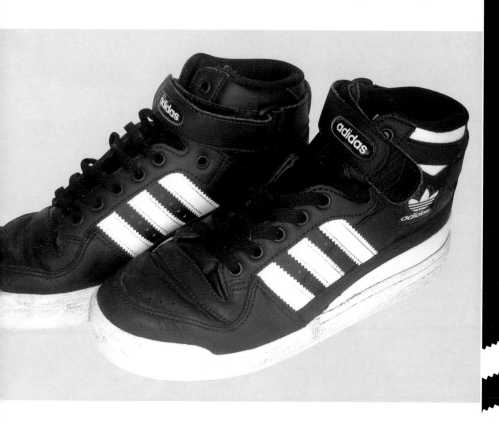

forum

The Forum is another famous adidas silhouette-shaped shoe and is probably the most famous and popular of all the adidas basketball shoes. They were built to last, with a tough leather upper to cope with the hard concrete street courts found all over the United States. Typically, adidas experimented with textures and the Forum was available in a shiny enamel finish, among other materials. The shoe came in Hi and Lo versions. But performance came at a price, and the Forum was one of the first models to break the $100 barrier in the U.S.

gazelle

The adidas Gazelle was launched in 1968 as an all-round training shoe and features a flat sole with soft velour leather upper. Seen everywhere in the world at some stage, and in a good range of colours, the Gazelle had a huge following among U.K. soccer fans. The pink version shown here is a rare example.

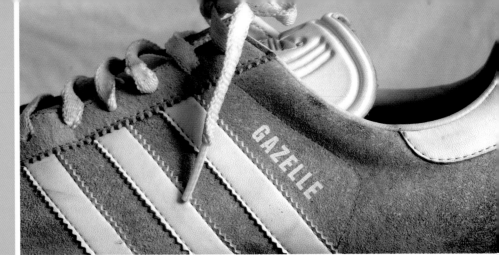

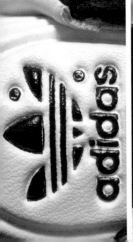

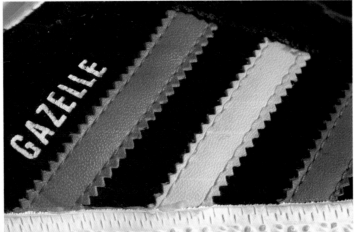

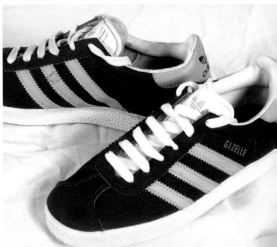

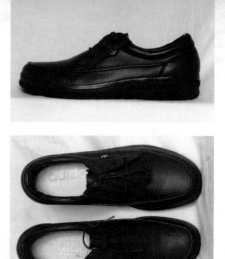

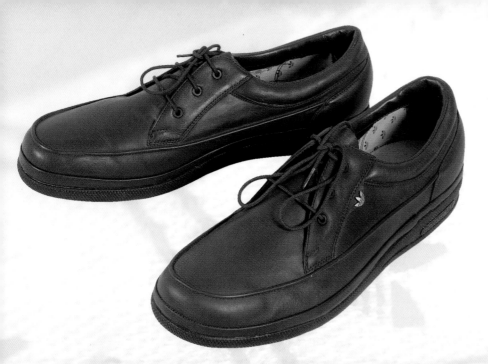

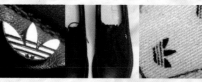

granada

This model is so shoe-like that it is questionable whether it should be called a trainer at all. It was released as part of adidas's official 'Leisure' series in the late 1970s/early 1980s, and all styles were picked up by the Casuals. The Granada is now an extremely rare model and has never been reissued to my knowledge.

handball spezial

The Handball Spezial was designed for ... you've guessed it! Handball. However, the Spezial was picked up by the Casuals, especially on trips to Europe. Therefore, it was common to see the German 'z' spelling on shoes in English-language markets. The shoes exhibit the silhouette and styling of the 'European Capital City' series of adidas shoes.

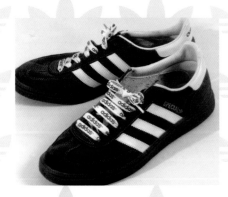

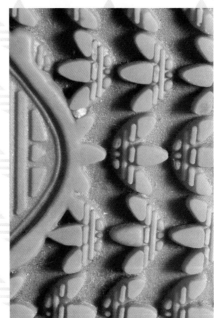

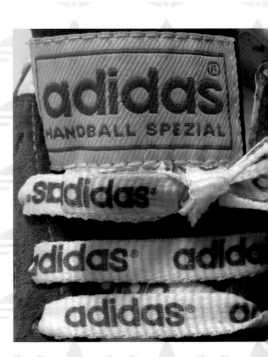

indoor match

The Indoor Match was a combination of a classic adidas canvas upper allied to a totally flat sole unit. The sole was especially designed for grip in order to stop squash and racketball players from slipping during their high-speed manoeuvres on the polished courts typical of this sport.

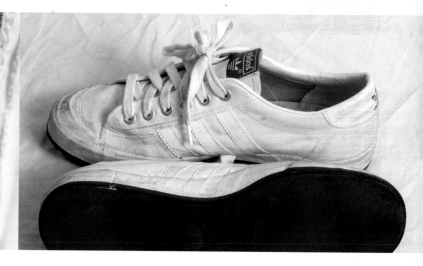

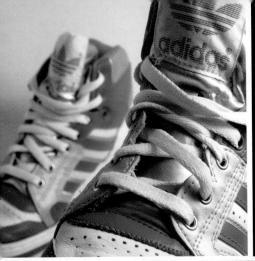

instinct hi

Adidas pushed back boundaries again with this basketball shoe. Hailed in the United States as the first 'streetball' basketball shoe, it was not for the fainthearted. Released in the early 1980s, the shoe gained respect with its advanced looks and strong performance, combining leather and PVC with crazy colours. As well as the colourway here, it was also available in red and gold.

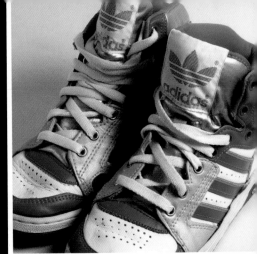

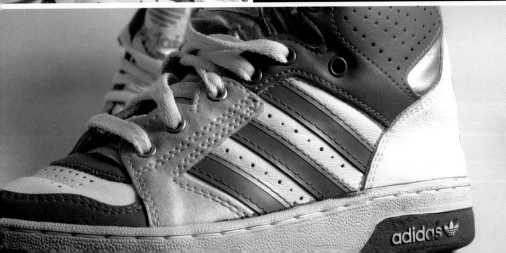

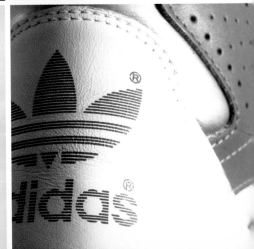

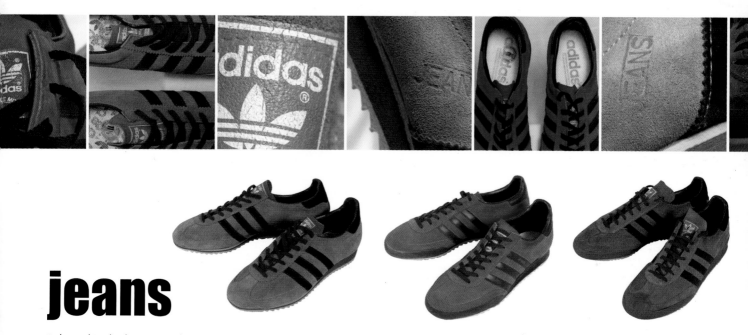

jeans

Released in the late 1970s the Jeans gained iconic status within the U.K. Initially developed by adidas under its 'Leisure' banner, the shoe was intended to be teamed up with jeans! Initially released in blue and red, later changes in design resulted in Jeans 2 and 3, but this model has never been reissued and so has retained its rarity appeal.

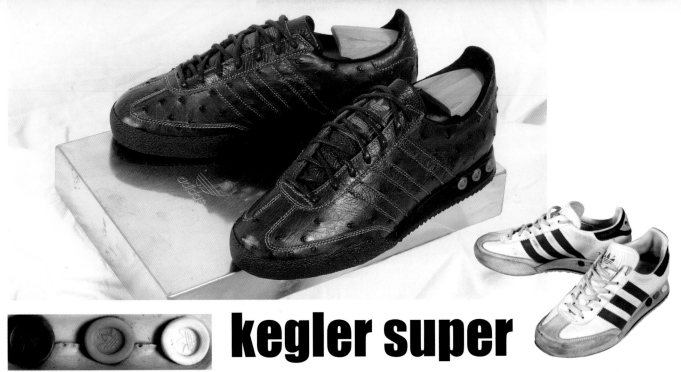

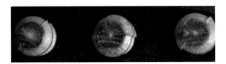

kegler super

Pushing the boundaries, adidas experimented with comfort and suspension with a series of models using its 'Peg System'. Found in the L.A. trainer and the Keglers, the system allowed you to use a series of moveable pegs to change the comfort or 'feel' of the shoe to suit your needs. The ostrich skin special edition seen here was a limited run of just 100 pairs, and was bought by a collector for £650 ($1,000).

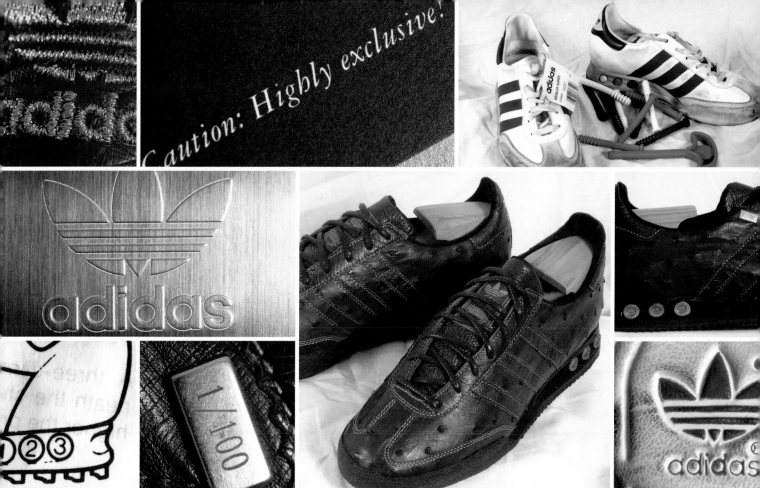

Caution: Highly exclusive!

adidas

1 /100

adidas

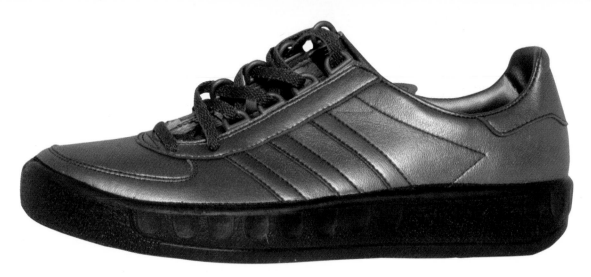

malaga

This is another of the 'Leisure' series of adidas shoes and dates from the late 1970s/early 1980s. However, this model sheds a little of the walking shoe vibe by exhibiting the classic signs of adidas tinkering with colours and materials. Even to this day, it's not too often that you would see a shoe with a shiny gold metal finish.

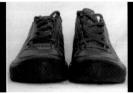

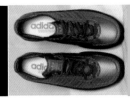

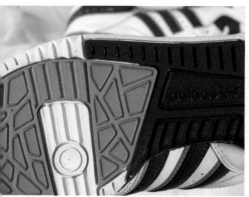

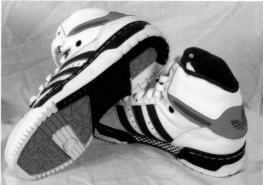

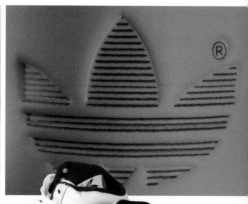

metro attitude hi

This is another shoe in the famous basketball series from adidas. The colourway here is in the livery of the New York 'Knicks' basketball team, and was particularly favoured by its famous player Patrick Ewing. Ewing eventually endorsed the shoe – his name was added to the tongue and so the Ewing model was born. The same shoe but without the orange at the heel becomes the Rivalry. The Attitude and the Metro Attitude are the same shoe in design, however the Metro has a snakeskin pattern that is picked out in one of the shoe colours.

mexicana

The Mexicana from adidas was an early forerunner of training shoes that have achieved far greater public awareness. This model has the silhouette of the Gazelle, as well as using the same flat sole unit and soft suede upper. Note, too, that this version features the older 'boxed' adidas style of lettering.

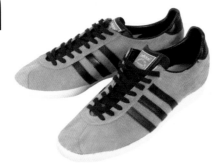

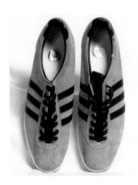

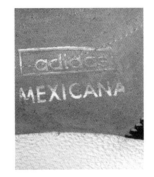

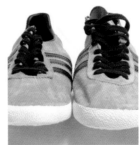

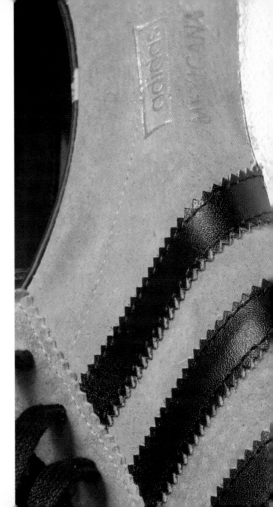

miami

Again, the Miami is an example of the 'Leisure' shoe that adidas developed over the years. These shoes were designed for comfort. Certainly not to everyone's taste, the design looks like it would be quite at home on your granddad's feet. However, attention to detail is crucial, and the tiny metal adidas trefoil is genius.

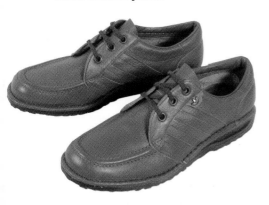

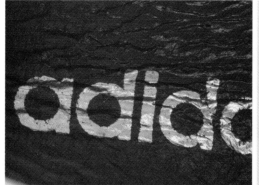

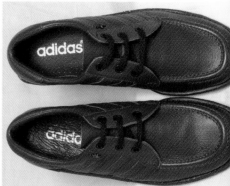

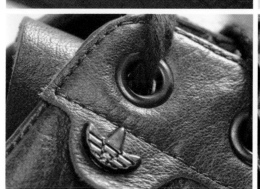

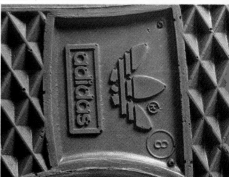

montreal

The Montreal was released in the early 1980s and is similar to the Centaur in terms of design. The model was intended to be a jogging or running shoe, but adidas just could not help themselves, and so made use of alternative colours just for the aesthetics.

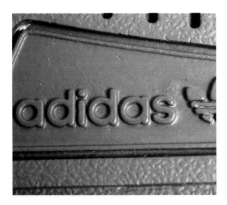

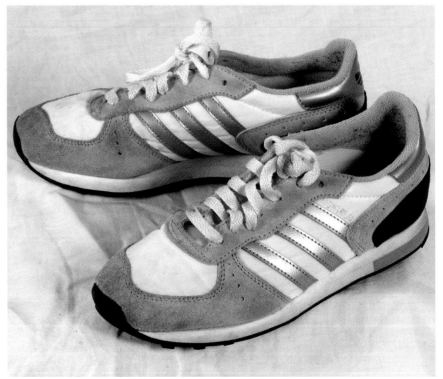

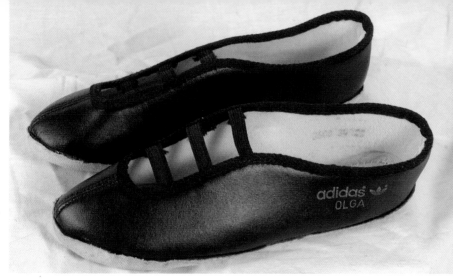

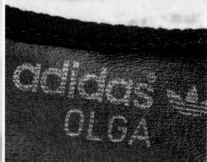

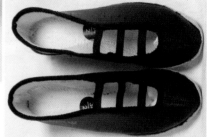

olga korbetts

This is another example of a sporting endorsement from adidas, but in a slightly less conventional design. The company produced these simple shoes as gymnastic slippers, made of Nylstretch – a form-fitting type of stretch nylon – with straps for a snug fit. They came in a basic black or white. However, in the late 1970s, when the young Eastern Bloc Olga Korbett dominated the world of gymnastics, adidas quickly snapped her up and put her name on the shoe.

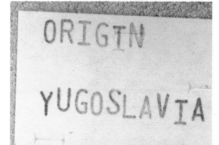

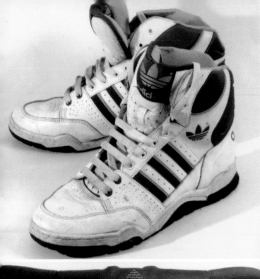

pro conference

The Pro Conference is an example of adidas's forays into the basketball market in the late 1980s. At this point, adidas was beginning to tone down the colours of its basketball shoes, and although the model was a developed version of its more famous brothers, the Instinct and Centennial, its quieter design generated less notoriety.

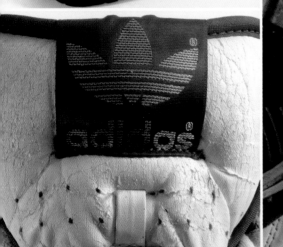

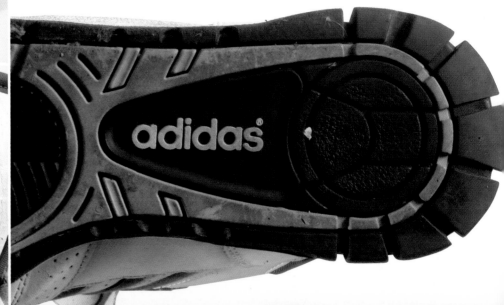

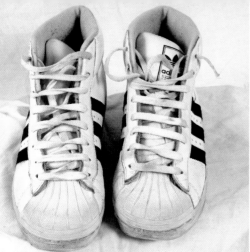

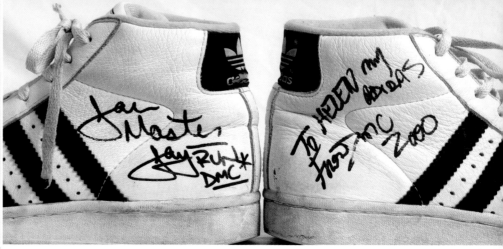

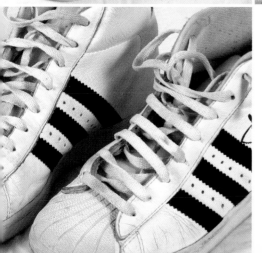

pro model

This classic adidas basketball shoe is basically
a hi-top version of the Superstar. The shoe was
released in the early 1970s but initially did not
feature the shell-toe cap. The early versions, made
in France, were leather and had the shiny gold label
on the tongue. They later went to a half-shell,
half-suede front and in the mid-1970s the shell toe
arrived. Later, the shoe was also made in suede.

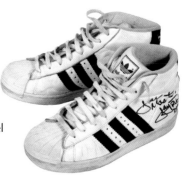

race walk

The Race Walk model was produced in the early to mid 1980s as a specialist shoe for race-walking athletes. Adidas exhibited confidence with its choice of colour on the design, though it was not a big seller at the time. The shoe is also available in a more conservative white with green stripes, but I think this one is vastly superior.

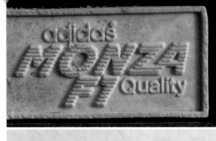

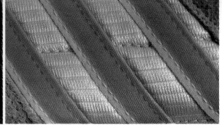

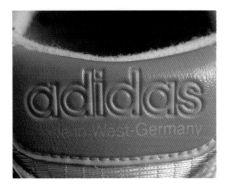

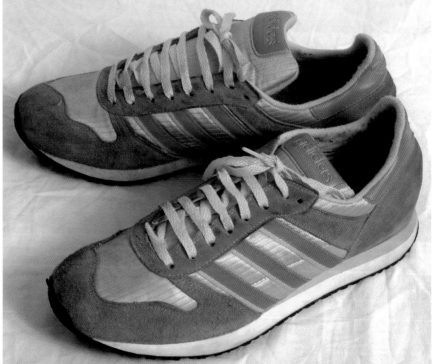

reno

The Reno is a particularly rare example from the 'Leisure' series produced by adidas, which has been comprehensively covered in this chapter. Typical of the series, this model exudes comfort. The series was also a radical departure from an emphasis on sporting performance and showed a move toward simple comfort and leisure. As usual, the Reno shows adidas employing quite daring colours to add impact. Along with the Malaga and others, this shoe was part of the 'Spanish' named series.

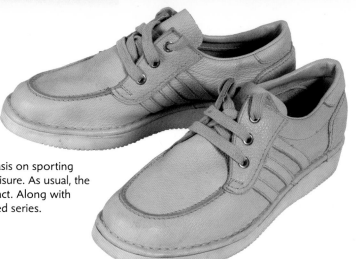

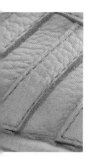
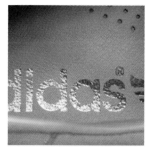
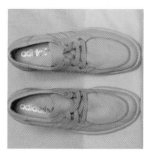
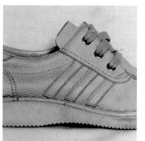
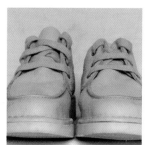
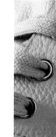

rod laver

The Rod Laver is simply one of the most popular tennis shoes ever. It was first developed in 1970 with the co-operation of Australian tennis great Rod Laver, who put his name to the model. The originals were in white with green and featured ventilated nylon uppers to increase 'breathability'. The model has found favour again recently, being reissued with all sorts of new colourways and materials.

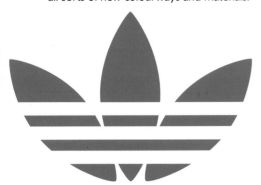

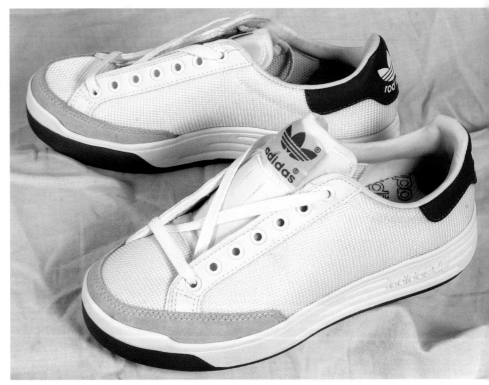

rom

The Rom was an adidas model initially released as a jogging shoe, and it utilized the same adidas silhouette as the Country. Although considered by some to be a simple design, it proved popular with the Casuals, especially in the north-west of England.

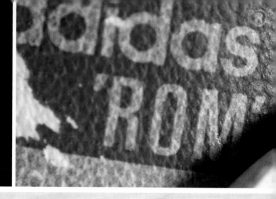

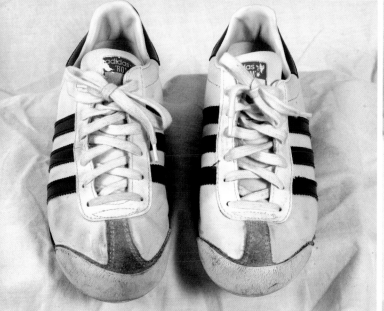

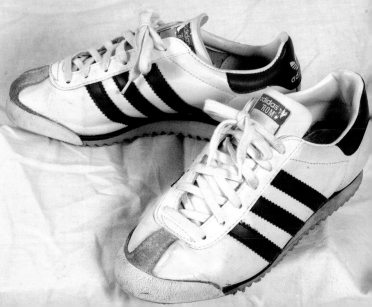

SL72

Launched for the 1972 Olympics (hence the 72 tag), the SL (Super Light) is a running/jogging shoe that was released in quieter, more subdued colours than its stablemate, the SL73. The 73 came in colours such as lime green or bright orange with yellow.

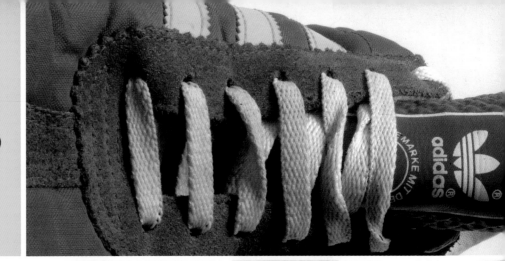

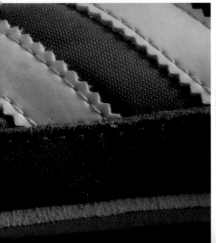

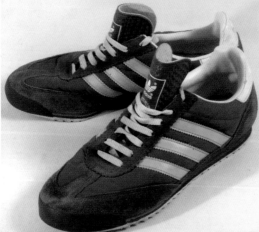

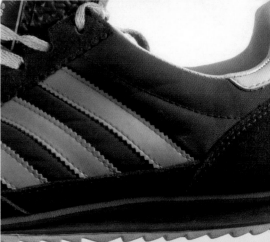

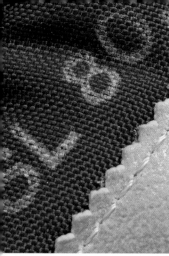
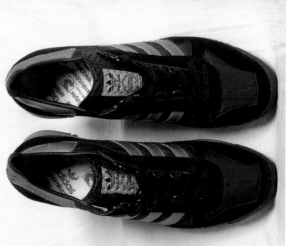
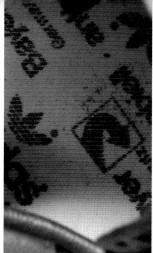
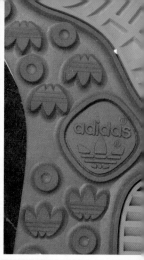

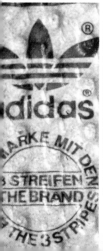
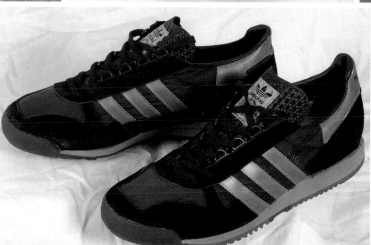

SL80

The SL80 model was released with a higher specification than others in the series, but it was essentially the same shoe, though it utilized more leather and had extra strengthening around the toe cap and heel. The 80 has the 'dimple' tongue and plastic 'ghilly' lace holes.

top 10 lo

Released in the early 1970s, the Top 10 is one of the oldest leather basketball shoes by adidas. It is an early shoe and so is basic, with a thin sole. It featured the basket hoop on the tongue and was an instant hit. Early versions, made in France or Morocco, are the most valuable. Due to its popularity, adidas produced the Lo version seen here.

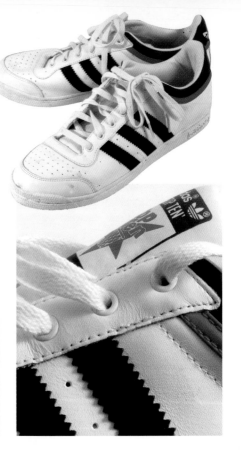

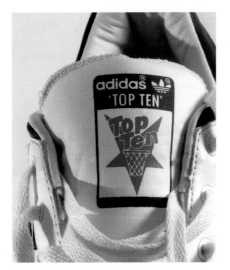

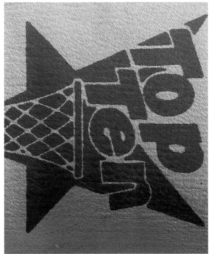

trimm master

This is another shoe that was designed for the fitness market from the adidas brand. The Trimm Master is not all that well known and is rare shoe indeed. Unlike its more famous younger brother, the Trimm Trab, the Master had a canvas upper and was made for indoor sports rather than outdoor track events.

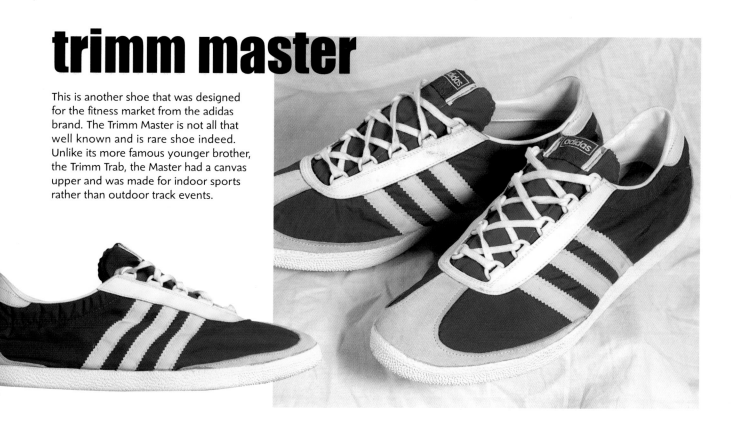

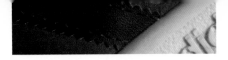
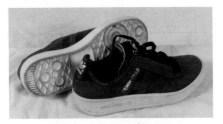
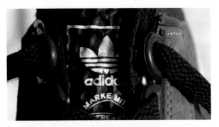
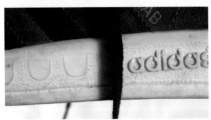
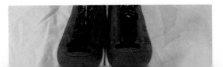

trimm trab

Loosely translated as 'keep yourself fit', fitness was the last thing on your mind when actually wearing these Trimm Trabs. They were released in the early 1980s as running shoes and became an instant hit with the Casuals. The indented polyurethane sole units are icons of an era of shoes associated with 1980s' soccer fans in the U.K.

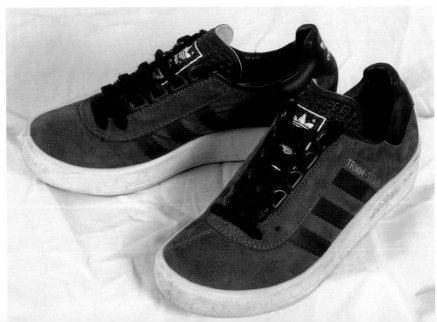

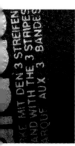
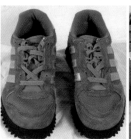
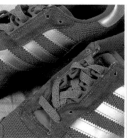
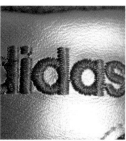
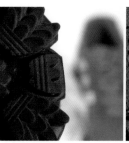
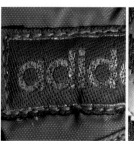

TRX comp

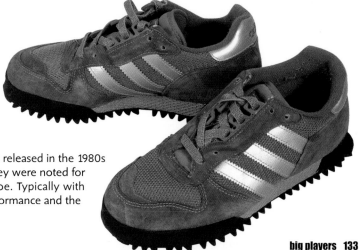

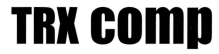

The Comp (Competition) is the top of the TRX series of shoes released in the 1980s and were intended for cross-country or off-road running. They were noted for their unusual soles, which overlapped the length of the shoe. Typically with adidas, where design is uppermost, style was allied with performance and the prominent sole was indented with mini trefoils for extra grip.

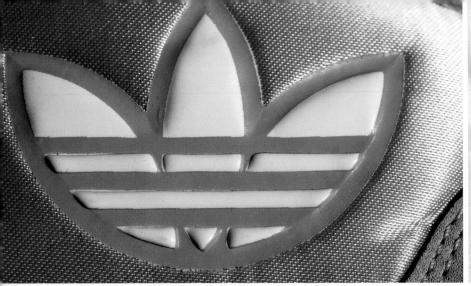

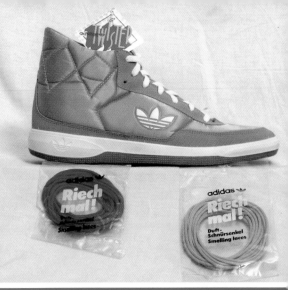

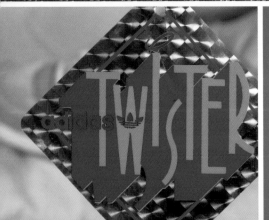

twisters

Released in 1985, Twisters combined strong design with outlandish colours and materials. With extra padding, the shoe was aimed at the developing Hip-Hop market. Available in shiny nylon in pink, yellow, sky blue, red and others, as well as hi, lo and ankle versions, they certainly made you stand out. An added extra was the inclusion of 'smelly' laces – literally colour-coded laces infused with various fruit flavours.

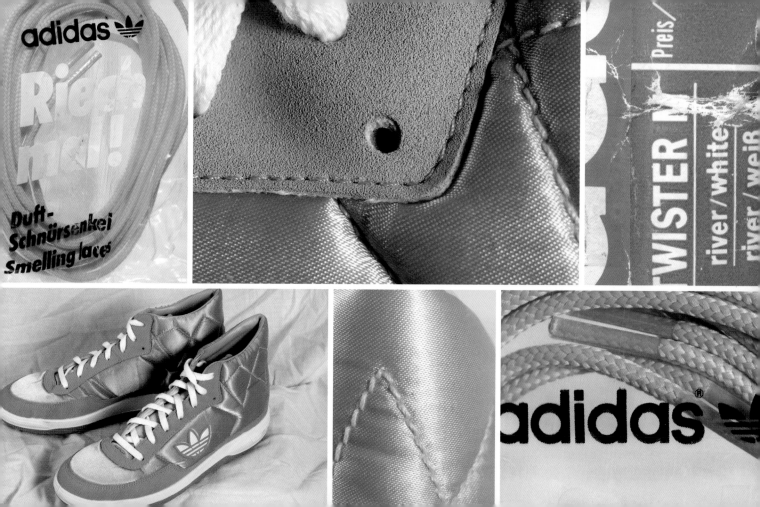

vienna

The Vienna is probably the oldest shoe photographed for this book, and it is an early example of an adidas design bearing the name of a European capital city. However, it is not one of the later City leisure shoes from this maker – instead of a suede upper we find leather, and the soles are too thin for comfort.

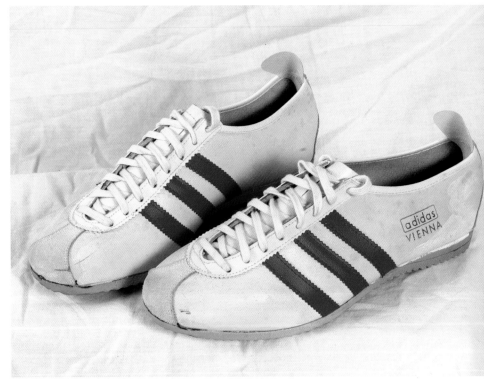

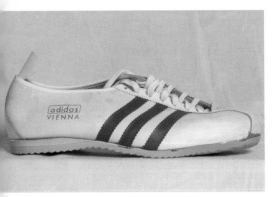

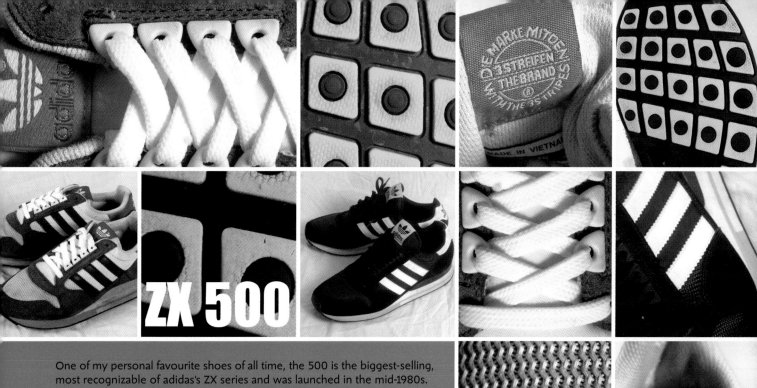

ZX 500

One of my personal favourite shoes of all time, the 500 is the biggest-selling, most recognizable of adidas's ZX series and was launched in the mid-1980s. The shoes were notable for their mix of technology and understated aesthetics. Typically the shoes were made from nylon and suede and utilized harmonious colourways. The 500 initially came in the light brown with yellow stripes version but it has been reissued recently in additional colours.

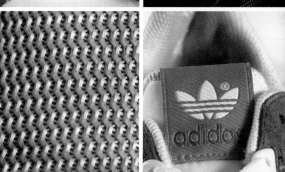

ZX5020

This member of the ZX series was very popular in the U.K. in the 1980s. It is a derivative of the earlier ZX500 with small changes in specification giving rise to different models The version here is in a garishly beautiful pastel colourway, and the model employs the 'Torsion' cushioning system so loved by adidas.

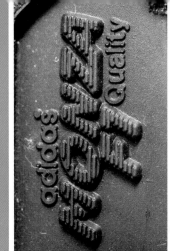

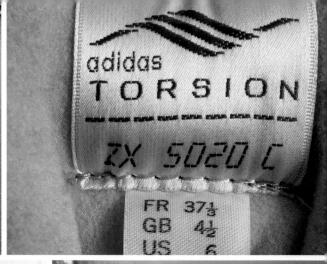

adidas TORSION

ZX 5020 C

FR	37⅓
GB	4½
US	6

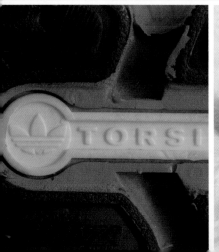

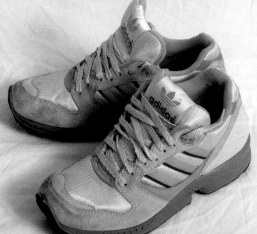

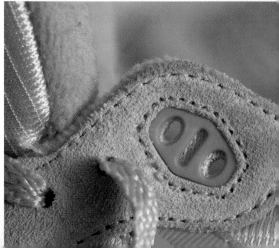

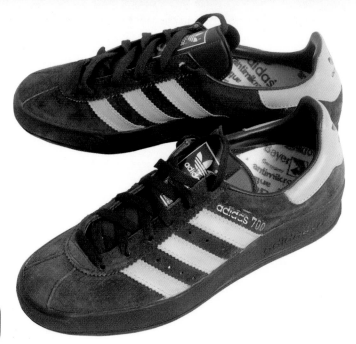

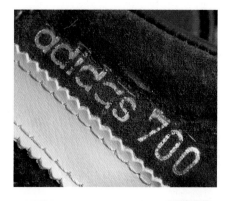

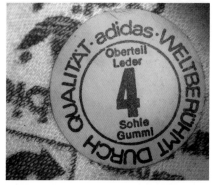

700

Developed as a running/jogging shoe, the 700 had one of the higher specifications of the '00' series of shoes of the late 1970s/early 1980s. Basically the higher the model number in the series, the better the specification of the shoe. At this point, adidas was paying a great deal of attention to aesthetics, and the 700, with its mottled tongue and studded-profile sole units, borrowed heavily from the TRX series.

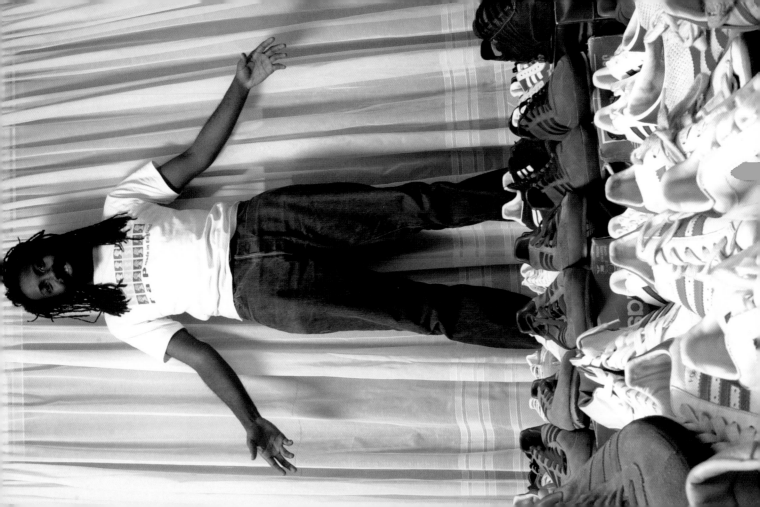

collector
ROBERT BROOKS

To anyone in the know, Robert Brooks is 'the man' when it comes to adidas. The 30-year-old graphic designer, born and bred in East London's Hackney, spent his formative years persuading his parents to buy him adidas ZX700, Forest Hills and Jeans. But there were many shoes that got away.

His craving for adidas trainers continued into his adult years and he began to build up a massive collection of rare, deadstock shoes. A well-known adidas aficionado with an encyclopaedic knowledge of adidas shoes and the brand, Robert supplied most of the adidas shoes photographed for this book. Robert has spent decades building probably the best adidas collection that I've seen. They are all here, rarities dating back to the 1960s: Jeans (3 pairs, all models); original Micro Pacers (2pairs/2 colours); specials such as the 'City' series; the runners; the tennis stars; and a pair of ostrich-skin Keglers in a gold box. Still searching, always finding, his passion is as big as his collection.

NH: Why this affinity with adidas in particular?
RB: I suppose it's on a few levels for me. First adidas had the best looking shoes, and timeless designs that were often way ahead of the rest. The running shoes were the ones: the attention to detail, quality materials, the use of 3M reflective material and the colour blocks in the sole unit. I strongly associate adidas with my youth and growing up. When I think of adidas I associate it with black cultural icons like Don

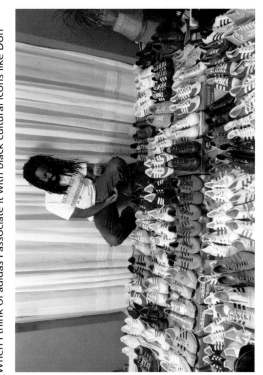

Quarrie, Bob Marley, Daley Thompson and Wilma Rudolph, whom the adidas Gazelle was named after. Adidas was the first brand I remember that supported black athletes.

NH: Robert, you have more than 200 pairs of deadstock adidas shoes and most of them boxed, is the searching a big part of it?

RB: Even when I was in school, and we went on school trips to France. We weren't thinking: 'Great, we're going to France.' We wanted to find the hot trainers, ones that you couldn't get in England. Of course, deadstock shoes don't fall into your lap. You have to seek them out, which adds to the thrill when you find something good. I persuaded a friend of mine, whose dad owns a sports shop, to let me have a look around his dad's stockroom in the hope of finding some deadstock adidas. He wasn't convinced that there was anything there. But I felt that there had to be something. Finally, he called me saying: 'Come to the stockroom, you won't believe what I've found.' I found a pair of adidas Jeans, a shoe I'd been searching for for years. But when we started exploring it was like 'OH MY GOD!' I found a pair of Roms, Mercury, Player and some other hot shoes. Also, boxes, it's the boxes. I remember a time when I went to Germany to buy trainers. I remember the guy taking us upstairs, and pushing open a door. And you know when you see that blue box? There were stacks of them, a wall of boxes, probably seven or eight feet high of blue boxes.

NH: Yeah, I know the feeling, I almost equate a lot of searching to 'the one that got away'.

RB: Yeah, at the time I didn't have the money to buy those shoes, I was too young. I wanted what my big brother had. I wanted to be like him. And then when you finally get what you want you feel sweet. It's funny, that now people are trying to buy into a culture that's been happening for years. It's not about how much you spend or how many shoes you have. For me, it's about memories, growing up in Holly Street Estate, hanging out in Dalston Methodist Youth Club wearing my adidas.

NH: For a while, all every article about trainers mentioned was what they were worth, how much they sell for on Ebay.

RB: Yeah, I get it all the time. People ask me: 'How much was that pair?' Or: 'How much is it worth?' It's worth only what someone's willing to pay for it! But to me the shoe's value is not linked to how much it can sell for. I'm only interested in the shoe, not how much I can get for it.

NH: There is too much hype around trainers today, from the teen mags right through to the style bibles.

RB: Yeah, it's like everyone wants a soundbite. If you go into a shop today, you might be able to buy a shoe for £60 and then sell it for £300, because there's been a limited edition release or a lot of media hype about it. Trainers are the thing of the moment so everyone wants to talk about it. I know what I like, which is why I spend time finding it.

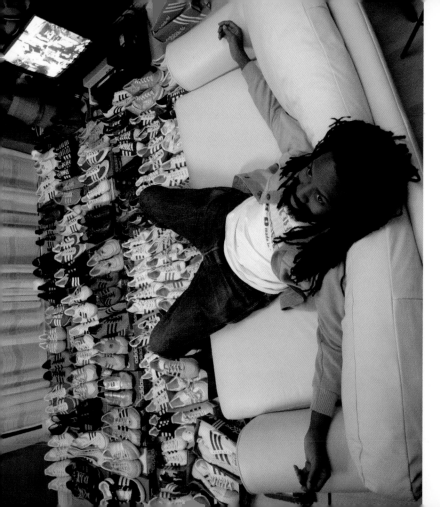

NH: I know it's hard Rob, but out of your collection what would you say is your number one?

RB: I don't have a number one, I have many favourites, Jeans, the ZX800 and the Micro Pacer. I remember when this shoe came out, I saw it in adidas Connection on Tottenham Court Road, London. For me, seeing that shiny silver shoe reminded me of an astronaut's shoe. People go on about adidas not being at the cutting edge of technology – it was 1984 and there was a computer in a trainer. The proof is in the shoe.

nike brand history

It was only 30 years ago that we had a world without Nike, and in that period Nike has gone from the brash newcomer in the trainer world to the number one mass-market leader. The Nike story begins with the meeting of its co-founders at the University of Oregon. It was here that middle-distance-running business student Phil Knight fell under the tutelage of the college athletics coach, Bill Bowerman. Nike would go on to grow out of the fusion of Bowerman's sporting innovation and Knight's marketing know-how.

It was in 1962, after Knight had been travelling in Japan, that the earliest business roots of Nike were formed. While travelling in the Far East, market-aware Knight had noted

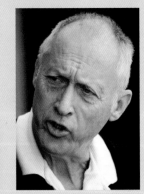

the production of training shoes that performed well and were competitively priced (in other words, cheap). The training shoes he especially picked up on were those of Onitsuka Tiger (a forerunner of the Asics of today). Utilizing his business-course leanings, Knight had the entrepreneurial idea of importing these high-tech but low-priced athletic shoes into the United States.

LEFT Phil Knight (far left) and Bill Bowerman, co-founders of Nike.

Interestingly, even at this early stage it seemed that Knight had a far-reaching goal – to break the long-established brand domination of the U.S. market by the then main player, adidas.

In order to achieve this aim, legend has it that Knight and Bowerman each put in $550 to cement their partnership, and decided to call their new company Blue Ribbon Sports (BRS). BRS was basically the American distributor of Onitsuka training shoes.

In 1965, after a period of selling Onitsuka shoes from the back of their van at athletic meets, the company grew. The first two full-time staff were added, both ex-college friends and renown track and field runners. These were Jeff Johnson and Steve Prefontaine (who left a job selling adidas football shoes).

During this time, the sporting half of the partnership, athletics coach Bill

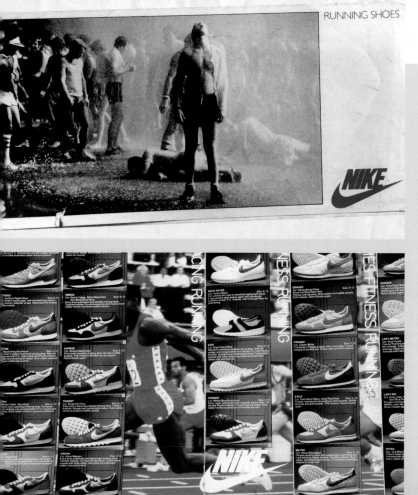

Bowerman, was constantly tinkering with the design of Onitsuka's trainers. In response to discussions with his track students, Bowerman's objective was to improve the performance of training shoes available to his athletes, and so ended up designing entirely new models, including the Marathon, Boston and a forerunner of the now legendary Cortez, the Corsair, for the Japanese shoe company.

The company went from strength to strength, but after heated disagreements between BRS and Onitsuka, the new boys at BRS decided to split from Tiger in 1971 and create their own company manufacturing their own shoes. But what to call this new company? It is said that Jeff Johnson came up with the idea for the new name, deciding to honour the Greek goddess of victory, and thus Nike was born.

It was also at this time that the fledgling company had to decide on a logo for the brand, and another of the legends that the company managed to create for itself was developed (*see page 147*).

TOP LEFT A mid 1980s Nike advertisement.
LEFT Running shoe catalogue from the 1980s.

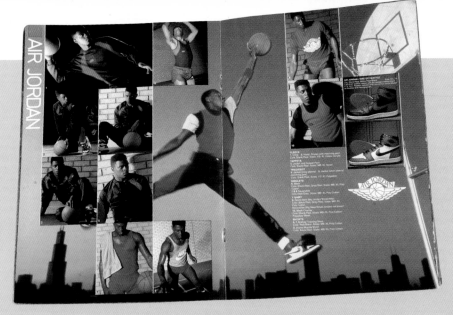

AIR JORDAN

LEFT A double-page spread from the original Nike catalogue devoted to the whole Air Jordan range.

At this stage, Nike along with its brand-new 'Swoosh' logo were released upon the world. Athlete and Nike employee Steve Prefontaine gave Nike its first public performance at the 1972 Olympics, with the most common question being: 'Who's Mike?' In this same year, Nike also produce the Cortez, the only shoe that has been continuously sold by the brand right up to the present day.

Nike took off virtually instantly in the United States, and within a year company sales were at almost 2 million pairs. Due to a policy of continuous product development,

the company kept growing and began to represent a serious challenge to the established companies in the marketplace. In 1981 Nike decided to take another major step, with the U.K. becoming the company's first wholly owned foreign distributorship.

However, it was in 1985 that Nike really became a major player. It was in this year that it managed to persuade the then little known Chicago Bulls basketball rookie Michael Jordan to endorse his own range of shoes. Even Nike could not have imagined the effect that this single act would have on sales. The new Jordan-endorsed range transported Nike and trainers in general to a completely new level of popularity.

It was after the introduction of the Jordan shoes and the mass-marketing that went

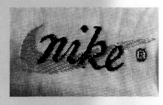 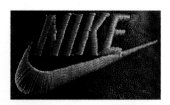 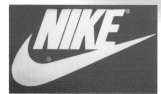 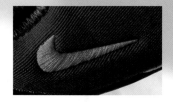

with them that the 'trainer wars' got underway. Each of the brands, desperate to stay one step ahead of the competition, came up with a continuous stream of developments and inventions of technical wizardry. For a while in the late 1980s Reebok actually overtook Nike to become the number one player (at least in terms of sales), but Nike came back strongly with its 'just do it' slogan in 1988, and regained the top spot in terms of market sales – a position they retain to the present day.

Nike has continuously pushed back the boundaries of trainer design, staying focused under Phil Knight's guidance, and is going to take some dislodging.

DEVELOPING THE SWOOSH

Back in 1971, the newly created Nike company was ready to hit the market with its shoes, and a logo to represent the brand was urgently needed.

Phil Knight turned to an associate from his teaching life and commissioned graphic-design student Carolyn Davidson to work with his new brand. Knight wanted a design that would represent movement. Davidson supplied Knight with a few designs, one of which was the initial 'Swoosh' so well known today. Knight was not particular enamoured with any of these designs, but with deadlines to meet the Swoosh was chosen. Knight admitted to Davidson:

ABOVE Evolution of the Swoosh logo (from left to right): 1971 version, 1978 version, 1985 update and the solo Swoosh from the 1990s on.

'I don't love it, but it will grow on me.' And grow it did.

Even though Davidson was initially paid only $35 for her design, the story doesn't end there. In 1983, Knight took Davidson out for lunch and presented her with a diamond-encrusted Nike ring, and also an envelope. The envelope contained Nike stock. We don't know how much was in there but a grateful Davidson will only state that she has been well compensated for her design.

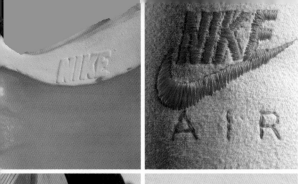

Released officially as the Air Force 180 in 1991 this is an underrated trainer classic. Nike took the 'Visible Air' design into new territory. In all honesty, it was aesthetics over performance, because once allied to the zingy colourways used, it became a shoe to die for! As the name implies, the 180 allowed you to see the air capsule from 180 degrees.

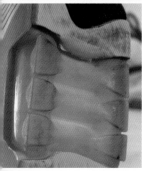

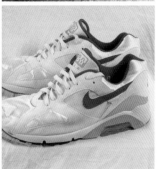

air
180

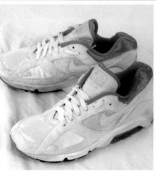

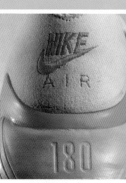

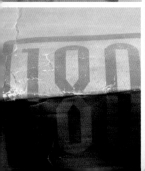

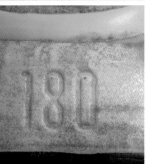

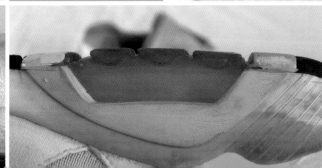

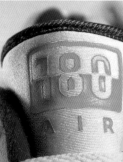

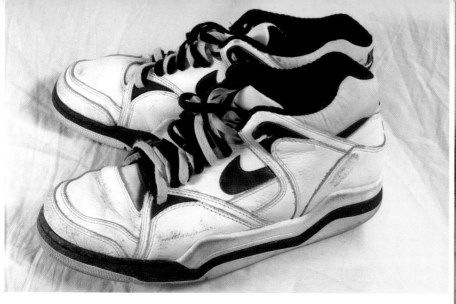

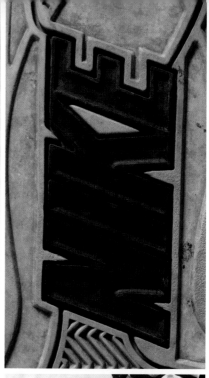

air bound

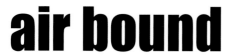

Released in 1991, Air Bound was essentially a mid-range basketball shoe. As well as designing to the edge, brands have to cater for all customers and budgets and the Bound was far more affordable than many others on offer. Ironically, due to its solid build and thick sole, the shoe became popular with ball players using concrete courts.

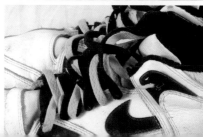

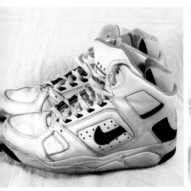

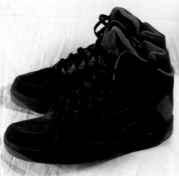

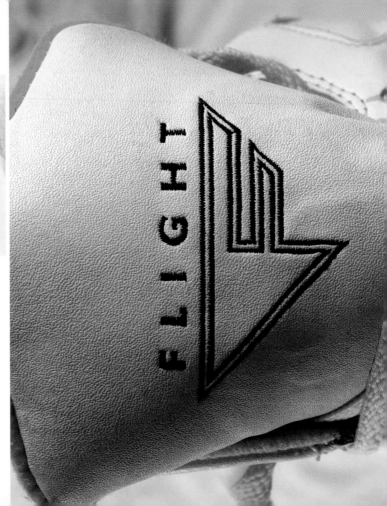

The original Air Flight Lite was released in 1989 as a basketball shoe and came in both Hi and Lo versions, The shoe also utilized the same sole unit as the Jordan 4 and was very popular with National Basketball Association players, such as Chris Marine and Tim Hardway. This later version didn't use the 'Visible Air' system found in the original Flight.

air flight lite

air footscape

Released in 1995, Air Footscape became an instant classic. The Footscape was released as part of the 'new wave' of trainer designs being produced by Nike. Like all design classics, it used a simple idea – in this case, the side lacing created a contemporary feel – and the shoe has been released in small numbers to maintain its appeal.

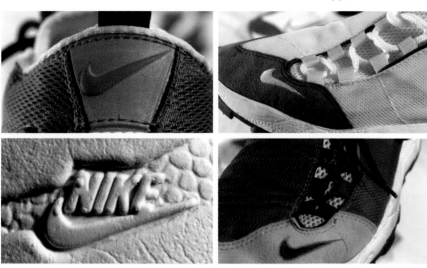

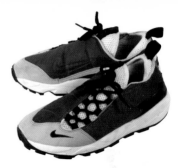

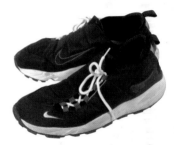

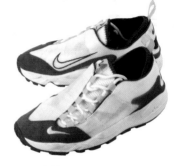

air force 1

This basketball shoe is such a classic it almost made it into the Hall of Fame. Released in 1982, it was the first basketball shoe to have full-length air inside the sole. Due to demand, the model has been reissued many times with slight variations and multiple colourways. The original colours, however, were white with red or royal blue or the rarer grey seen here.

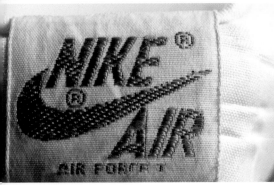

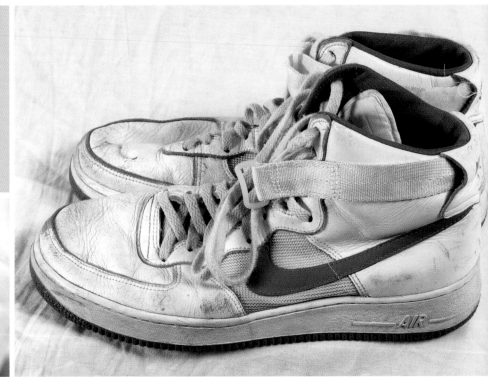

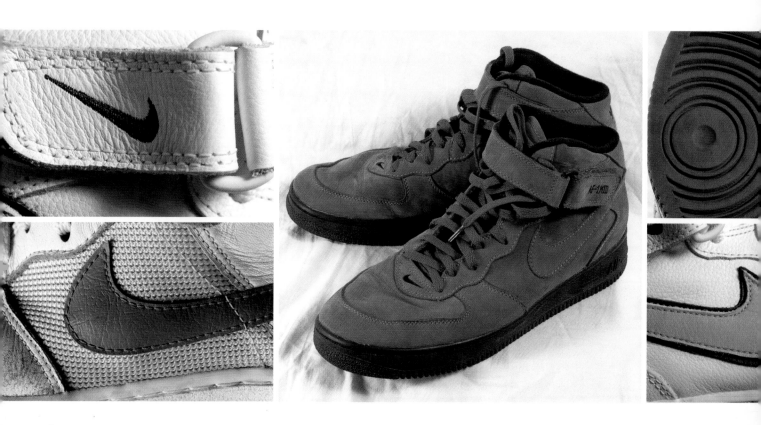

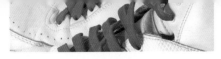

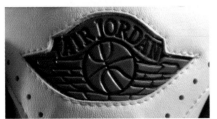

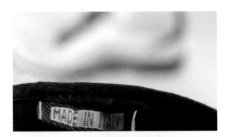

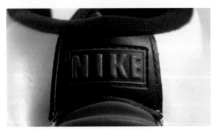

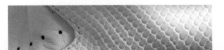

air jordan 2 ▶

Released in 1987, the Jordan 2 was designed by Georgio Francis and Bruce Kilgore and looks unique within the Jordan series. Sometimes referred to as the Italy Jordan, after its country of production, the 2 was the only Jordan not to be made in a black version. It was also the last shoe of the series to exhibit the original 'Winged Basket' logo.

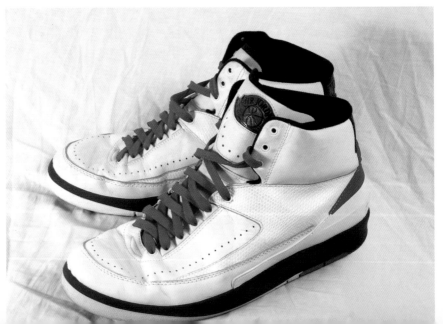

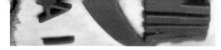

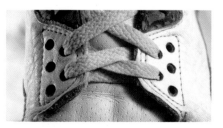

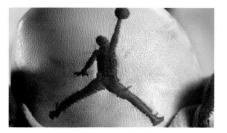

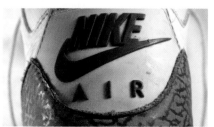

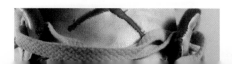

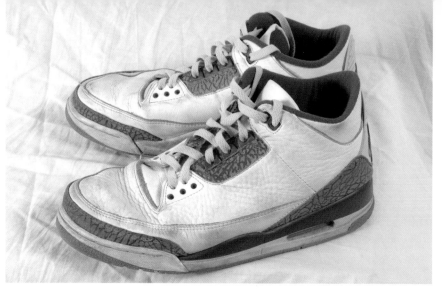

air jordan 3 ▶

The Air Jordan 3 was released in 1988 and is probably the most popular shoe of the series. It featured a number of firsts. It was the first Jordan shoe designed by Nike legend Tinker Hatfield, who went on to design all the Jordans up to 15. It was the first Jordan to exhibit the 'Jumpman' logo, and it was the first to utilize the 'Visible Air' sole units. This model regularly wins 'Top shoe of all time' polls.

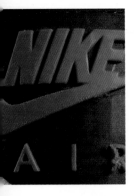

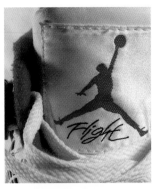

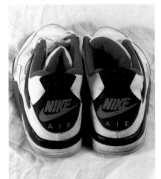

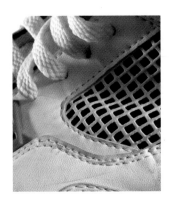

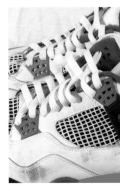

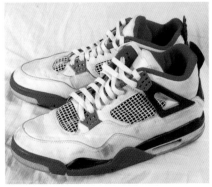

air jordan 4 ▶

The next Hatfield-designed Jordan, the 4, was issued in 1988 and was based heavily on the 3. One obvious change was the 'Flight' logo on the tongue, and it's the only Jordan to use it. Due to the popularity of wearing shoes with the tongue turned down, Air Jordan labels were sewn inside the tongue upside down so they could be read from above. The model also has plastic hoop shoelace rings inspired by basketball hoops.

air jordan 5 ▶

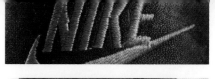

The Air Jordan 5 was released in 1990 and has the dubious distinction of being the first shoe that someone actually killed for. It is said that Hatfield was inspired by the 1940s' Mustang fighter plane, and this can be seen in the 'shark teeth' shapes on the side of the sole. The 5 was also the first shoe to use the clear-plastic sole unit, which enabled the 'Jumpman' logo to be seen inside. It also featured the 'lace-lock' system.

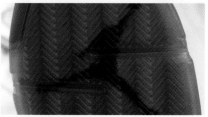

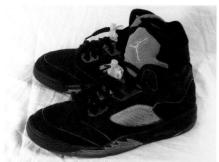

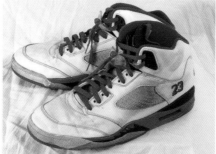

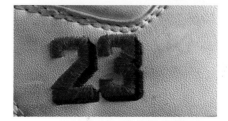

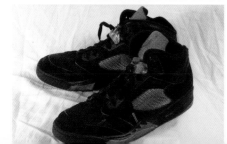

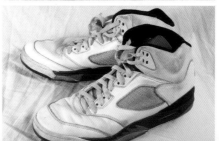

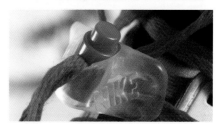

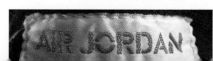

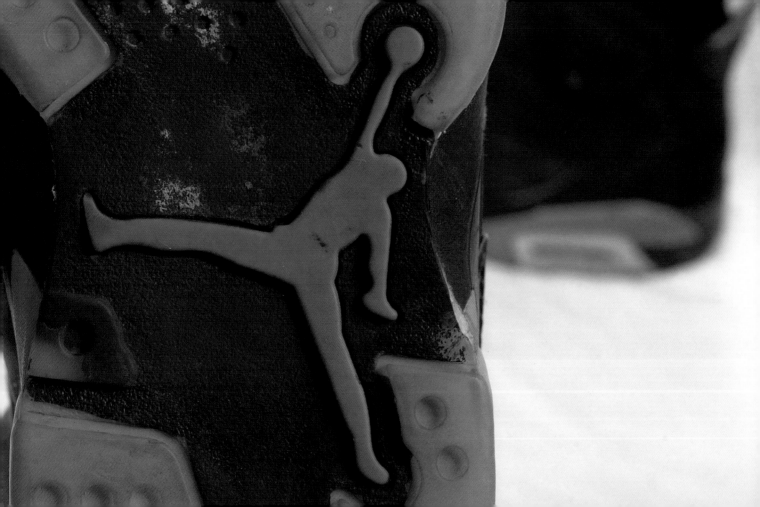

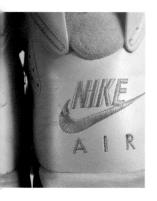
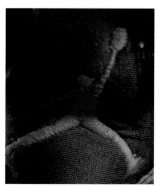
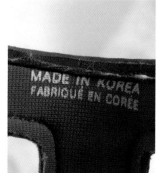
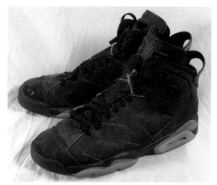
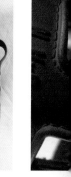

air jordan 6 ▶

The Air Jordan 6 was issued in 1991 and it was the last of the Air Jordan series to feature the small 'Visible Air' window in the sole. The model is said to have had some air flow problems, something that prompted Michael Jordan to cut an extra air hole in the shoe's toe. The model is notable for its use of hook holes in the tongue, which made it easier to put the shoes on.

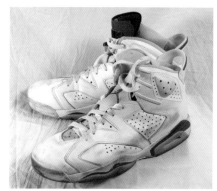

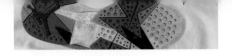

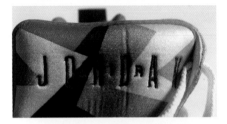

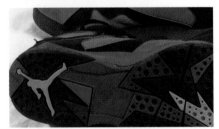

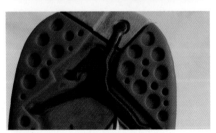

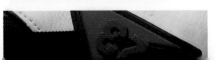

air jordan 7 ▶

With Jordans increasing in popularity, Nike upped production. The 7 was released later in 1991, looking similar to the 6, but included an inner sock to increase comfort and fit. This was the first Jordan that didn't use Nike's 'Swoosh' logo. Also, Jordan's playing shirt number, 23, no longer used on limited editions, became standard on all Jordans.

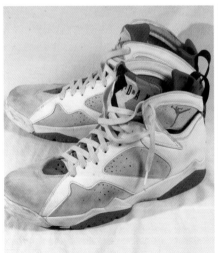

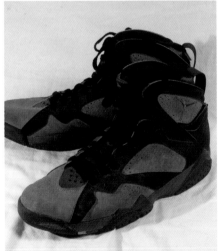

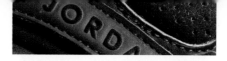

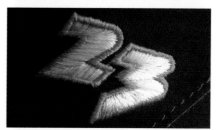

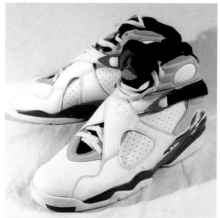

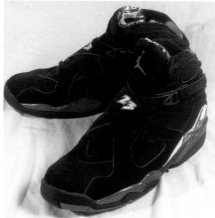

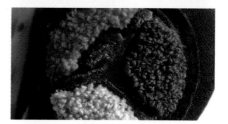

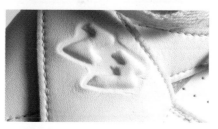

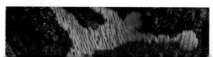

air jordan 8 ▶

The Air Jordan 8 was released in 1992 and demonstrated a significant change in Jordan designs. The designer, Hatfield, took inspiration from Nike's Air Raid, and employed the same 'cross-belt' system, intended to hold feet tightly in place, in the Air Jordan 8. The 8 was released in only three colourways – black/red, white/red and black/blue – apparently in an attempt to control sales.

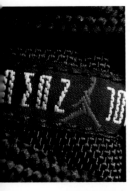
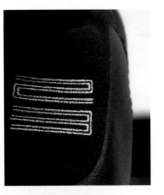
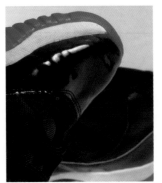
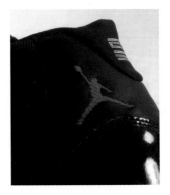
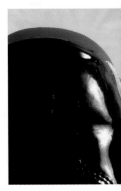

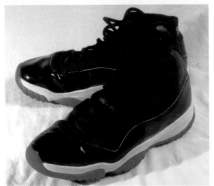

air jordan 11 ▶

The Air Jordan 11 reaped the benefit of years of Jordan-buying mania in a big way.
By the model's issue date in 1996, the hype surrounding the shoe had been fine
tuned to such a degree by Nike that on its initial release the Air Jordan 11 became
the fastest-selling shoe of all time. This model is always to be found in magazine
and internet 'top polls'.

air jordan 12 ■

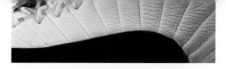

The Jordan 12 was released in 1996 and, to be truthful, I think it is an ugly-looking shoe. It has been featured here as an example of the new trend in 'space-age' shoes that have been giving trainers a bad name. However, it's all personal taste and lots of people do like them. Here, an extra-large size has been placed next to a standard size.

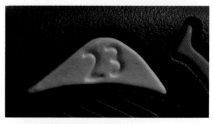

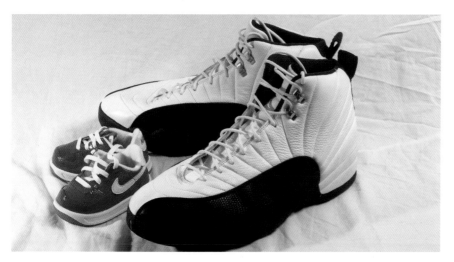

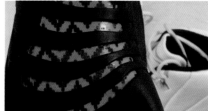

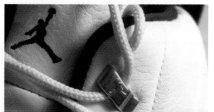

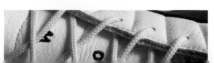

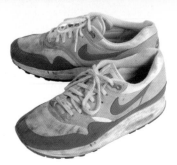

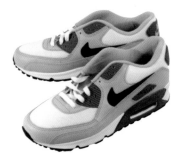

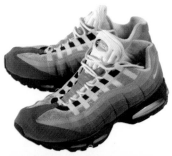

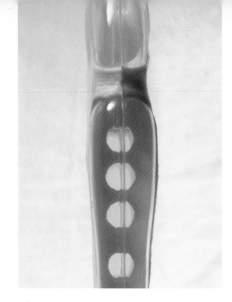

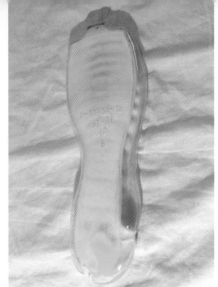

air max 1, 90 & 95

The Air Max 1 and 95 shoes have already featured in the Hall of Fame, but the other model here is the Air Max III, which is commonly known as the Air Max 90 (after its year of release), and it is a reissue with a new colourway. The 'Air' phenomenon has left an indelible mark on trainers. It is a simple idea and was developed brilliantly with the 'Visible Air' windows – a feature taken to extremes with the Air Burst and 270.

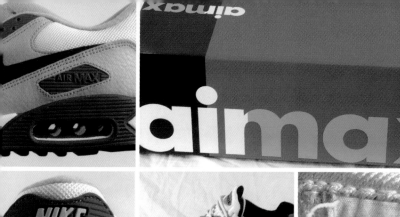
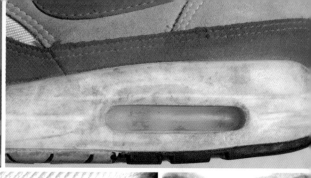
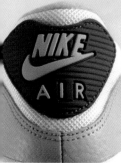
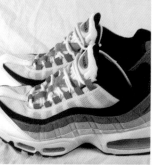
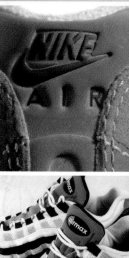
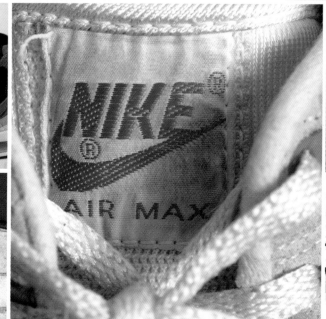
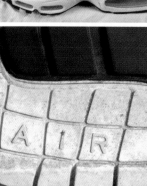
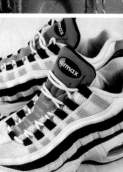

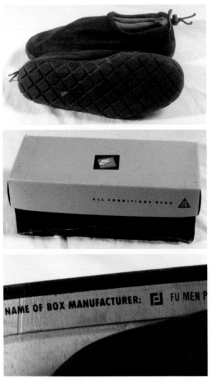

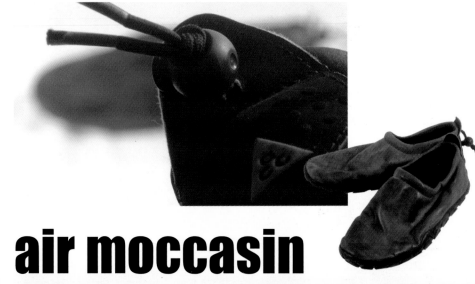

air moccasin

Released in 1994, the 'Air Moc' as it is more commonly known, was one of the holy trinity of style-changing shoes (along with the Max 95 and Footscape) Nike released in the mid 1990s. The Moc was part of the ACG (All Condition Gear) range developed for 'outdoor adventures'. It combines old with new in a bizarre mix: the upper has the look of a moccasin, while the sole unit is very thick and robust.

air mowabb

The Air Mowabb was released in 1991 and it is one of the most underrated models produced by Nike. The shoe came out with the ACG (All Condition Gear) series and was a highly specified walking or mountaineering shoe. Some versions included the Huarache 'inner sock' system, and I am certain that these are destined to be a future collector's item.

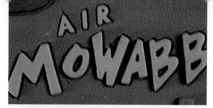

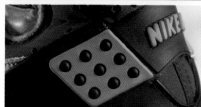

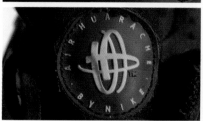

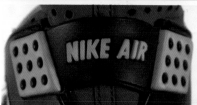

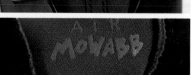

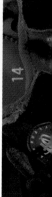

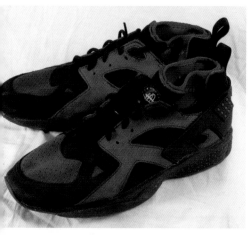

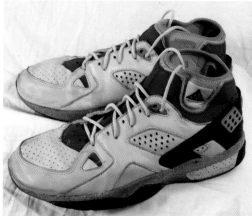

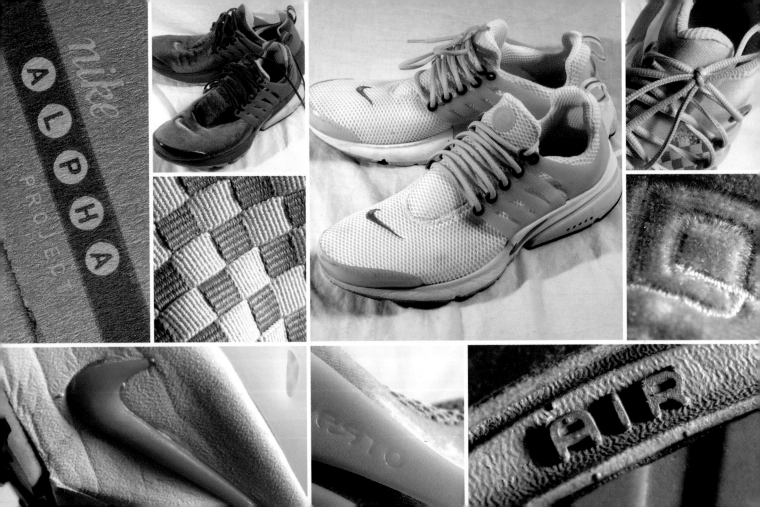

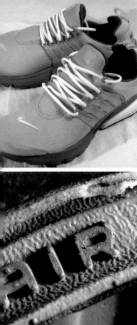

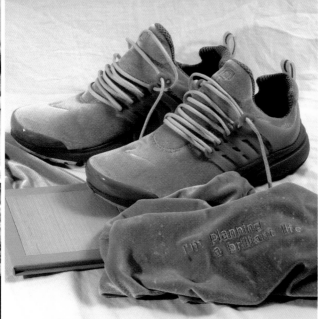

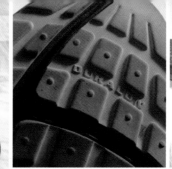

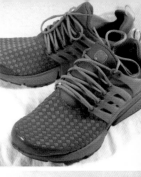

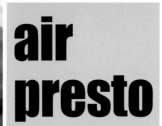

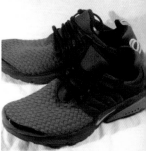

air presto

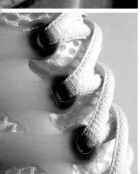

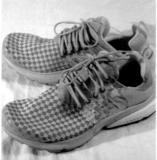

Just as you think there's nowhere else to go, Nike pushes back the boundaries. Released in 2000, Air Presto is a shoe that will be looked back on as a piece of classic design. It took a 'classic' design shape and fused it with modern materials and concepts. Nike's running shoes seem to be linked to its basketball shoes – as good as the runners get, the baskets get uglier. The versions seen here include variations such as the Presto Woven and Presto Suedes.

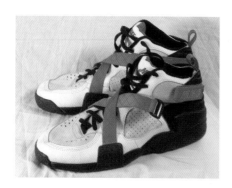

The Air Raid model was released in 1992 and was intended for the 3-on-3 type of basketball, with soles designed specifically for outside use. The model is known for being the first to use the cross-strap system, developed to aid fit. The model came in many colourways, some developed for specific stores – the one here is the Athletes Foot livery.

air raid

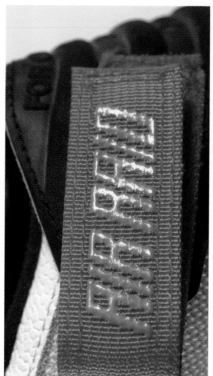

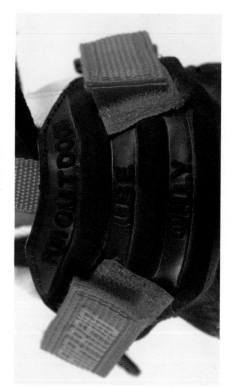

air raid peace

Released in 1993, these shoes were officially called Air Raid II but are more commonly known as Peace. In an attempt to move away from the 'conflict' associations of the Air Raid name, Nike developed this model with its messages of harmony on the rear and a peace sign on the cross strap.

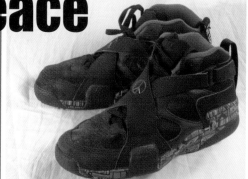

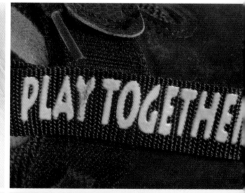

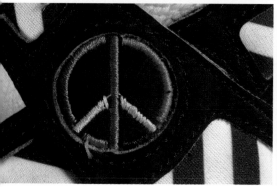

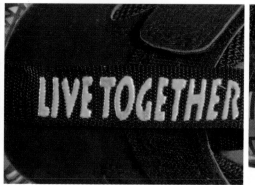

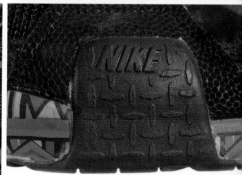

air rift

These shocking shoes were released in 1996. They were developed for the Kenyan running team, who traditionally ran barefoot and liked the fit of split toes (the Green colourway is the Kenya official colours). Nike also took inspiration from the Japanese Ninjas, who wore split-toe boots similar to this. Onitsuka were making split-toe trainers in the 1950s for the Japanese market.

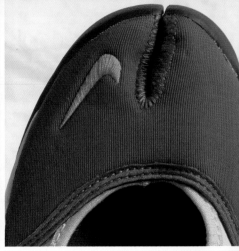

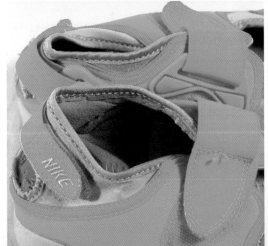

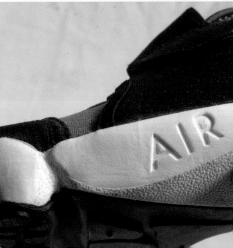

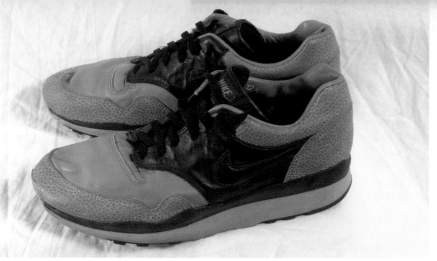

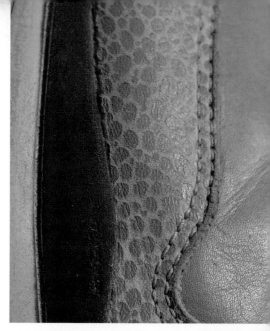

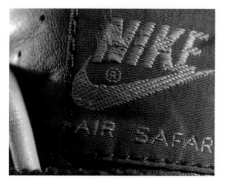

air safari

This Nike shoe is gaining 'underground' support before its reissue. The Air Safari was released in 1986 as a running shoe but it did not attract particular acclaim at the time. It was in the mode of the Air Max 1 in shape, but it did not utilize the Air Window design. In keeping with its model name, the Safari used artificial leopard and snakeskin material.

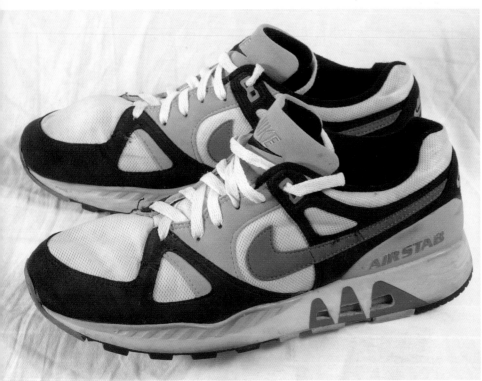

air stab

The Air Stab was released in 1988 and was officially a part of the 'Air Max' family – running shoes with the air-sole unit on display via the Visible Air window. The straps over the footbridge were intended to 'develop motion' and control ability. Personally, I think this feature, allied to the partially concealed window, spoiled a good piece of design.

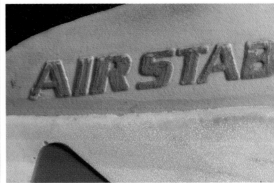

air tech challenge

The Air Tech Challenge model – or the Air Agassi as they are more often known – was released in 1988. The shoe gained its name when tennis champion Andre Agassi came on board with an endorsement. It was at the same time that the crazy colourways the shoe comes in were developed to match the colourful tennis champ himself.

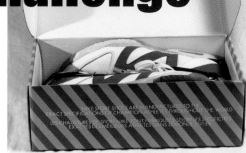

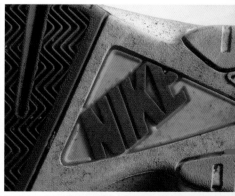

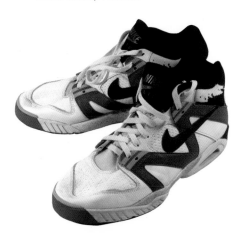

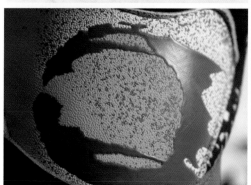

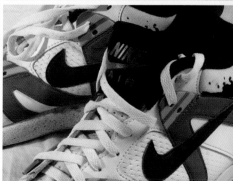

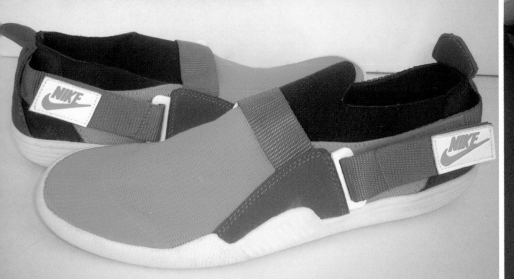

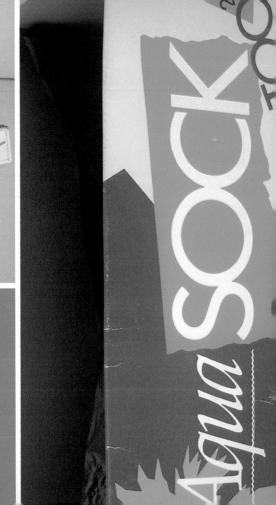

aqua sock

The Aqua Sock was an innovative idea from Nike. The shoes were intended for water sports, such as surfing and boating. They are a lightweight model made with a mesh upper designed to allow the water out. The sole is tough for walking in water on rocks. The shoe was released in 1985 in the United States and in 1990 in Europe. The bright colours of the shoes matched those of the box.

blazer

The granddaddy and the oldest of all Nike basketball shoes, the Blazer was released in 1973. Its aim was to knock adidas and Converse off the courts. The initial Blazers had a particularly large Swoosh logo and were available in leather, suede and canvas. There is nothing groundbreaking in its design, but this shoe helped to launch a giant.

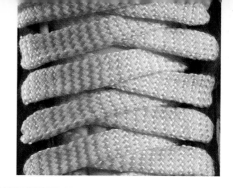

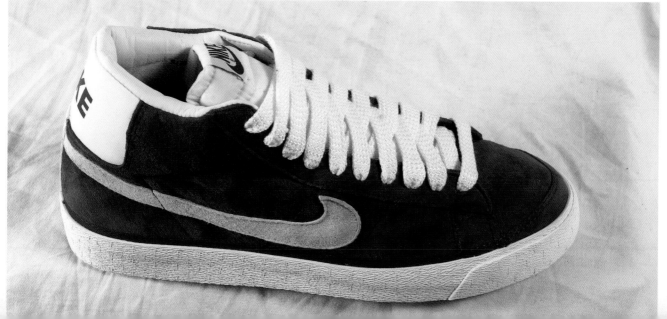

bruin

The Bruin is another of Nike's oldest designs and is a legend. Released as a lo-cut basketball shoe in 1973–4, the model is very similar in design to a Blazer Lo. However, the Bruin was released in many different colourways and was noticeable for its thick rubber sole incorporating a herringbone pattern for better grip.

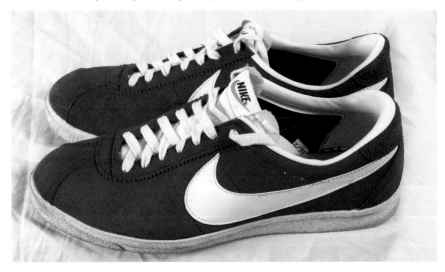

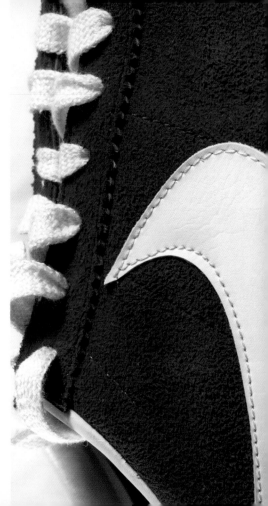

cortez leather

Not only is the Cortez one of the first shoes ever made by a then fledgling Nike company, it also has a history with the Japanese manufacturer Onitsuka. More importantly, the shoe is the only model that Nike has continuously produced since its establishment back in 1972.

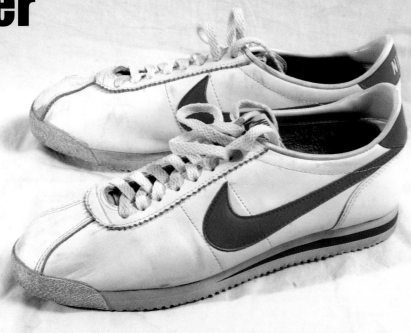

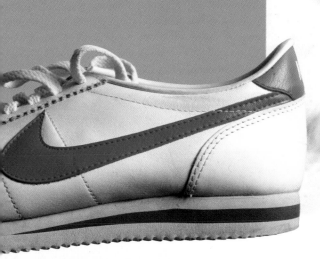

delegate

The Delegate was released in 1984 as a specialist tennis shoe, but it exhibits two features that are not normally associated with Nike products. First, it used cross straps in place of laces and, second, it replaced the applied Swoosh logo with an outline of the famous symbol in perforated holes.

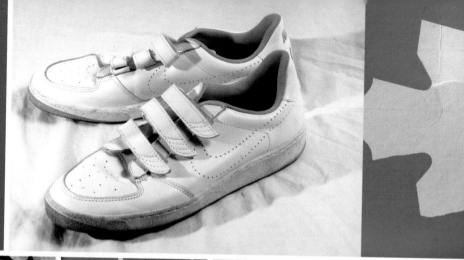

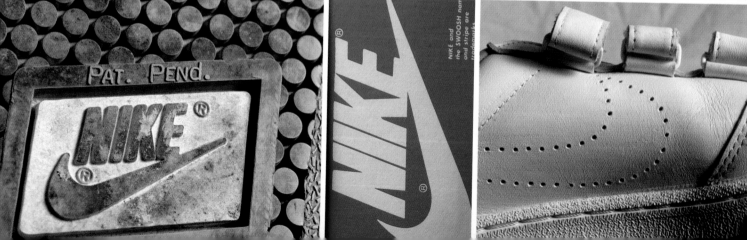

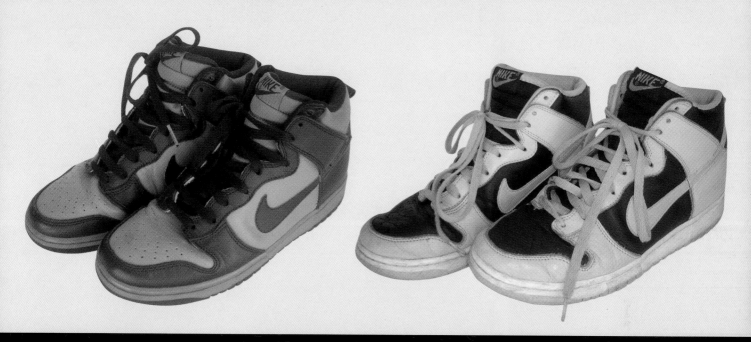

dunk

The Dunk was released in 1986 and its multiple colourways immediately caught the imagination of the American market. The shoes came in hi and lo versions and also had two sets of laces to match either shoe colour. They were not initially released in Japan, but it was there that fashion lovers made the shoe the cult object it is today.

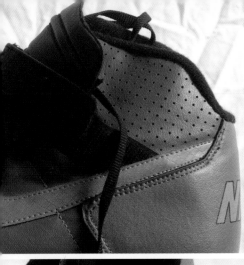

fatz

The Fatz model was released in 1988 and was intended for cross-country and similar types of running involving rough terrain. It had a stiff sole, not unlike the Lava Dome walking shoe, and also a leather covering for the lace area that could be strapped down with Velcro. This feature was designed to stop mud or water getting into and clogging up the laces.

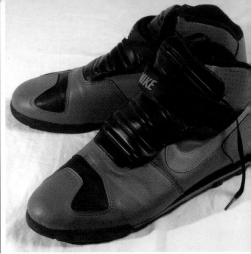

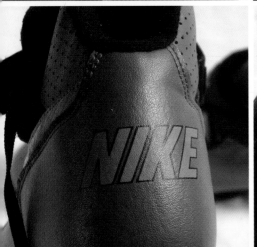

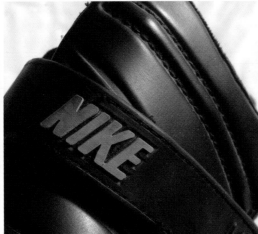

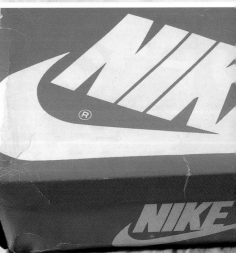

huarache

In 1993 Nike released its Huarache series of trainers. There was a basketball version as well as the normal runner (seen here in white), and the super-lightweight, higher-specification Huarache Racer (here in blue). The new idea was an inner sock worn inside the shoe with the shoe cut away to expose the ankle, and a reinforced forefoot providing extra stability. People liked them, especially the Racer, which gained many fans.

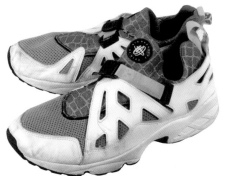
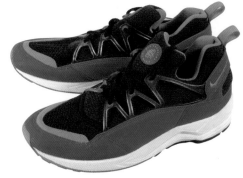

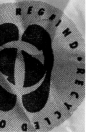
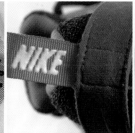
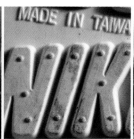
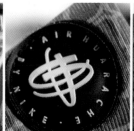
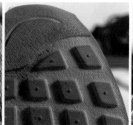
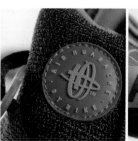

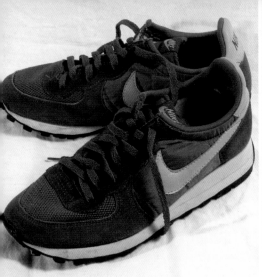

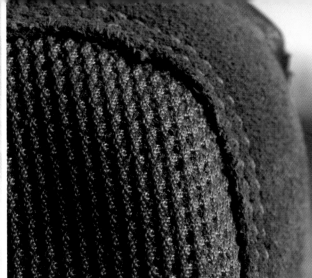

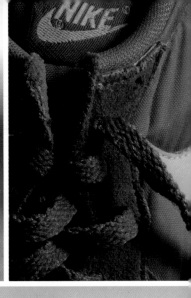

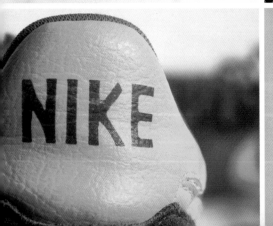

internationalist

This classic Nike running shoe comes from an era when many people feel that the company was at its best. The Internationalist was released in 1982 and exhibited the classic shape seen in many shoes of the same era. It was one of the first Nike shoes, along with the Wimbledon, that was picked up and adopted by the Casuals in the then adidas-obsessed U.K.

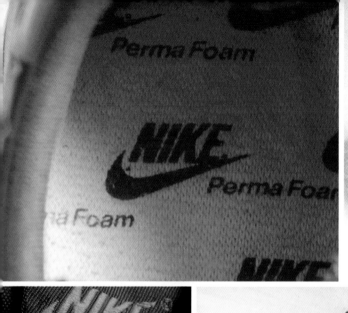
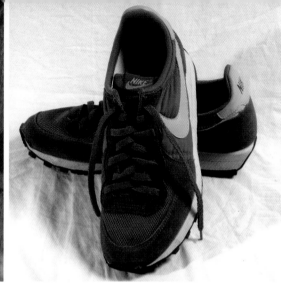
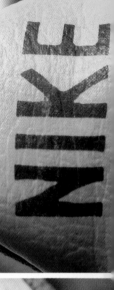
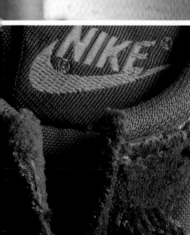
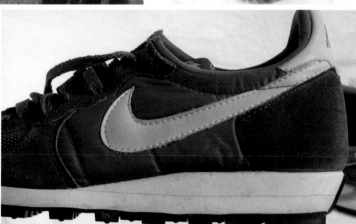
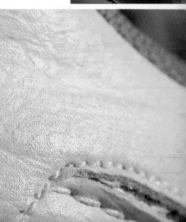

lava dome

Nike's Lava Dome was released in 1989 and it was a very early attempt by the company to produce a walking-cum-mountaineering shoe. Later, the Dome range of shoes was developed for the ACG (All Condition Gear) range, which was released in the early 1990s. The Lava Dome was very robust in construction and with little flexibility. To increase its appeal, Nike brightened up the walking world with its use of lurid colours.

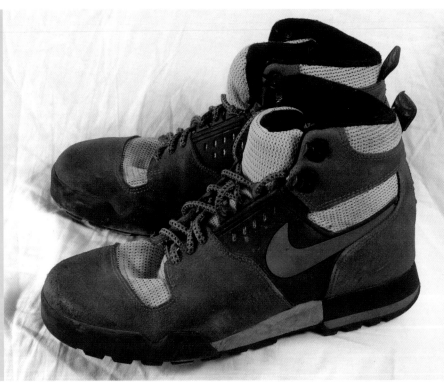

omega flame

The Omega Flame was released in 1983–4 and was a spin-off design of the already established Omega series of shoes. Not particularly heralded at the time, and not really well known outside the inner circle of Nike fans today, this shoe is definitely a well-kept secret. The Flame name is reflected in the use of a diffused colourway of flame-type colours employed in the Nylon upper.

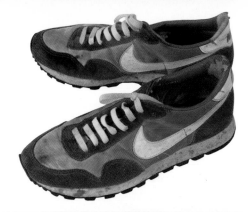

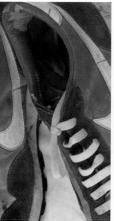
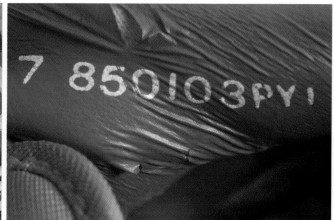
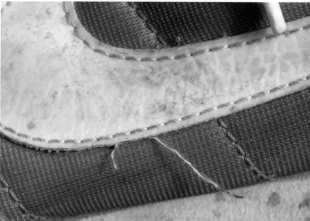

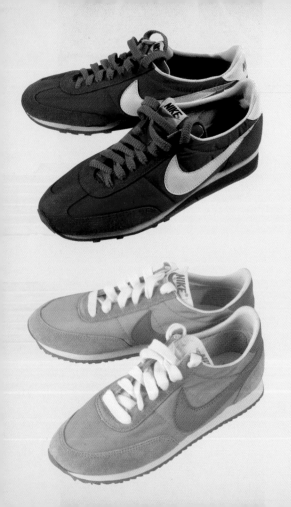

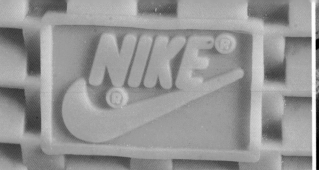

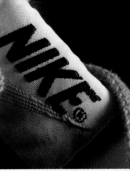

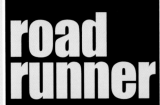

road runner

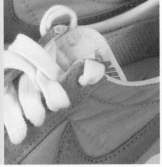

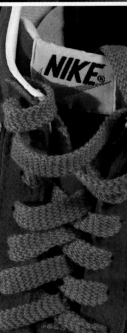

The Road Runner is probably one of the most famous of Nike's nylon running shoes from the late 1970s. The Road Runner was released in 1976 and it seemed that every Nike shoe looked similar to this until the mid 1980s. There was also a female version, the Lady Road Runner, which usually came in softer pastel colours.

scout

The Scout is a lesser-known example of a Nike running shoe dating from the 1970s. It was released in 1977 and this style of trainer was all that was seen from Nike for some time. Look closely and you will easily spot this style of trainer in many films and detective shows from the late 1970s.

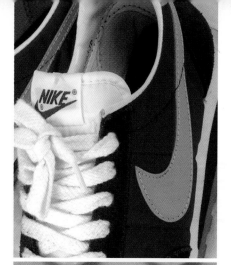

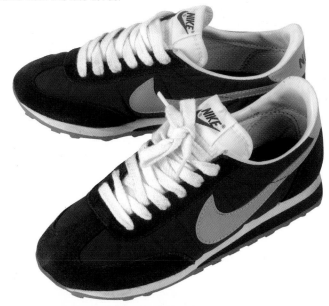

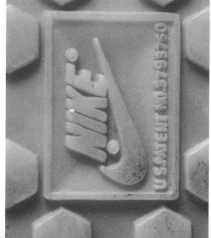

terra t-c

The Terra T-C was released in 1982 and continued the tradition of classic Nike running shoes, such as the Roadrunner and Scout, from the late 1970s. There was nothing groundbreaking in the look of the T-C, but its design and colourway ensure an appealing product.

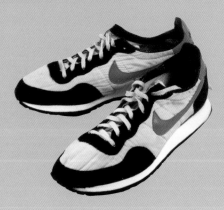

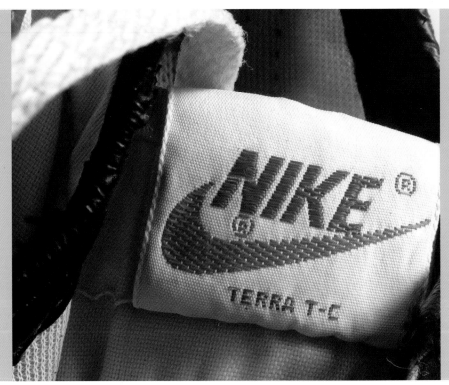

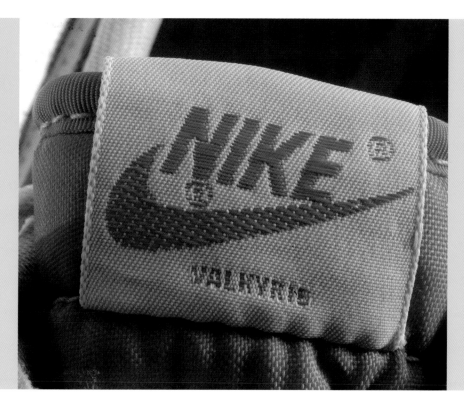

valkyrie

Like the Terra T-C opposite, the Valkyrie is another simple yet classic running shoe from Nike. Although it was released in 1982, the Valkyrie is reminiscent of many Nike runners from the previous decade. Note, too, that this shoe is from the era when Nike included the name of its models on the tongue.

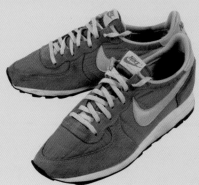

vandal supreme

The Nike Vandal Supreme, first released in 1987 at the top end of the series, has just been re-released and is generating a lot of interest. These shoes had always been bright, using heavy canvas in red or green with a gold Swoosh, but the Supreme took the colours to another level with shiny silver material and brightly coloured ankle straps. Too garish to be a big success at the time, the shoes are now part of Nike folklore.

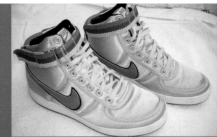

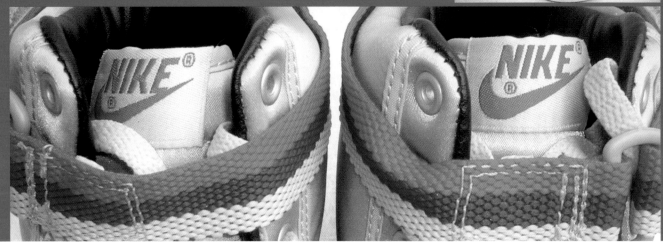

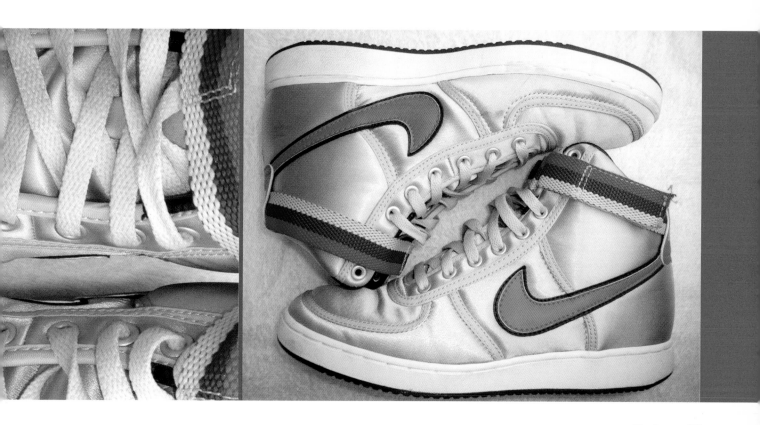

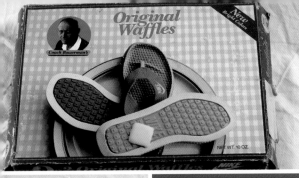

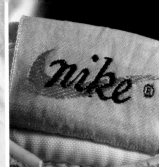

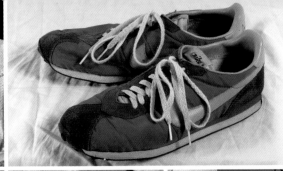

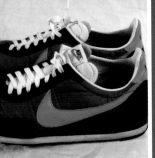

waffle & waffle racer

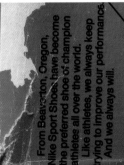

These are two of the most famous of all trainers. Worn in the early 1970s by runner Steve Prefontaine, though not released until 1974, legend has it that Nike was inspired by the pattern on a waffle-iron when looking to improve the sole units for the shoes.

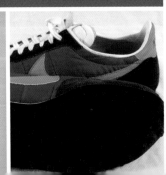

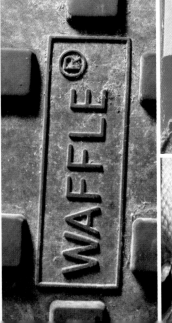

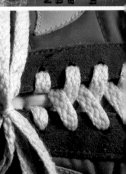

194 big players

wimbledon

Designed as a tennis shoe, this classic model had been made by Nike for some years in various guises and under different names. But when the new kid on the block, John McEnroe, wore them at the famous lawn-tennis championships in England in 1979, the Wimbledon name was adopted for the shoe.

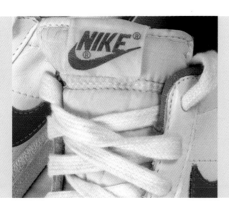

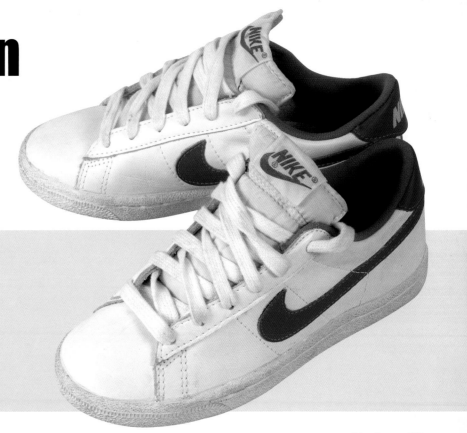

collector
JEREMY HOWLETT

In a room like an Aladdin's cave to a deadstock hunter like me, I sat and talked trainers with Mr Nike, better known as Jeremy Howlett. Jeremy has over 3,000 pairs of the Swoosh branded shoe, and his knowledge of the brand rivals that of Mr Knight himself. Jeremy kindly supplied most of the Nike shoes photographed in this book, and his enthusiasm is hard to describe – we could have filled this book with his thoughts.

'I lived in a small English town and got into trainers through skaters. I really loved the image of such early skate guys as Tony Alva we saw in the early days of skate in California. Alva and the rest of the Z-Boys always seemed to be in Nike Blazers and they struck a chord with me.

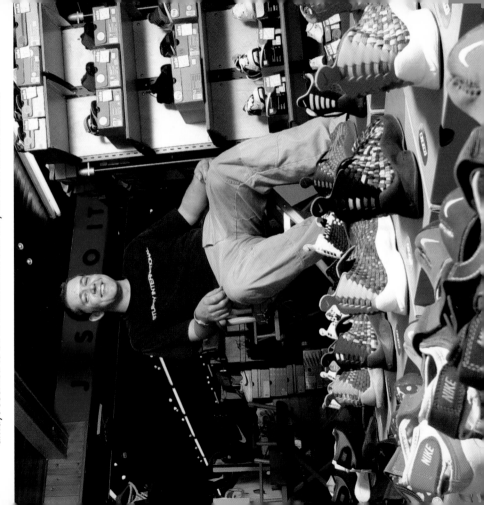

So when the family went on a holiday to America I bought a load of the early Nikes. This would have been around 1974 or 1975. Nike was a small concern at this time and it had only a limited range of footwear really. Either you could have a shoe in a lo version or the same shoe in a hi version. The models I saw around then were Blazers, Bruins and of course Cortez. But it was the Bruins that stuck with me.

When we returned to the U.K., I persuaded my dad, who owned a sports store, to try and import this new brand – not with any foresight, but just cause I loved the shoes and wanted them for myself and friends. But Nike were so small then, nobody was selling its shoes in the U.K. and there was no distribution process. In the end, we managed to source a Californian tennis store that would sub-order for our store, and this is how we started to import early model Nikes into the U.K. I really think that hardly anyone else was doing this in Britain at the time. Maybe Soccer Scene up in Carnaby Street, London, but that's it.

So, amazingly, probably the best kitted-out Nike wearers in England were from a sleepy seaside town. We used to go up to London most weekends and skate the Thames Embankment or go to the Brentford Rolling Thunder Skate Park. This is where the other kids used to see our shoes and really wanted them too. A friend and me started working in the Alpine Sports store, in the City of London, because they sold skate stuff, and we started taking orders from kids who saw the shoes we wore and wanted them, too. I ended up being a courier, as my dad would order the shoes for these kids from the shop and I would then deliver them up to our mates in London.

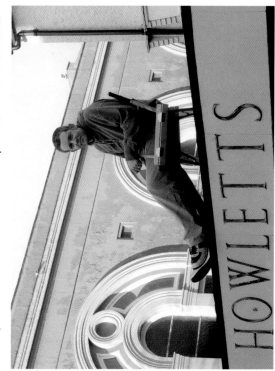

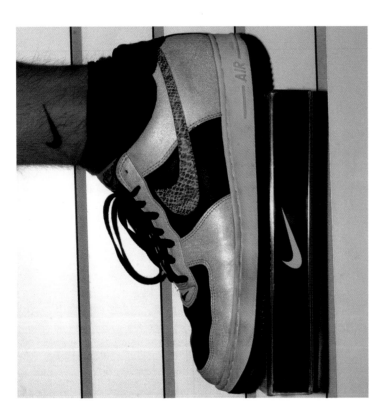

This was a bit easier then – from about 1979 a small company in Newcastle started importing and distributing Nike in the U.K. and we could get our stock there.

However, it wasn't until around 1982 that I think I really got into the collecting habit with Nike shoes. It was then that the Nike range took off and they offered a much wider variety of shoes. Also, John McEnroe won Wimbledon in his Nike Wimbledons this same year, and it was then that Nike really entered into the mass consciousness of the U.K. public. In particular, the football Casuals used to come into the store and buy the Wimbledons, when they had not bothered with Nike before. So it was then I started what you could call collecting. It wasn't a conscious decision along the lines of "now I'll start", I just loved the shoes, the brand, and wanted the new models as they came out. In this way, my collection started to grow.

To be honest, I have an obsessive personality – whatever I'm into, I'm really into. I love records so I have a huge record collection. I didn't choose collecting, it chose me This may sound mad, as I have more than 3,000 pairs of Nikes, but I have never been a Nike collector as such. If I was a real collector I would never wear the

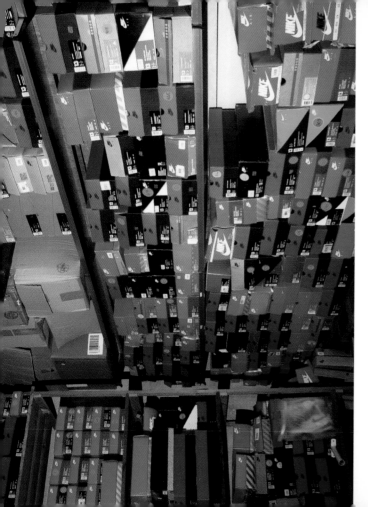

shoes. And I never buy the shoes to trade, so I don't buy all models. I only buy the trainers I like a lot. For instance, when rare issues or limited-run shoes are released, I don't get lots (which I could easily do). Instead I buy myself maybe two pairs, and I wear them both. A lot of people would buy loads of them for reselling. I have to love the shoe to buy them.

If I had to choose my top five shoes of all time then they would be: Air Jordan 3 (there is no other); Rifts (I just don't care if fashions come or go, I love them and always will); Omega Flames; Blazers; and finally there is Bruins.

Even though the Air Jordan 3 is my favourite shoe of all time, I never really got into the Jordan phenomenon. I love them, but I think it's more of an American thing really, particularly a Black American thing, and it has gone around the globe.

I think the thing is its easy to become jaded and cynical with trainers and that's why I try to keep the unjaded attitude of people who are fresh to trainers, such as my wife, Karen. If she likes a shoe she will simply wear it. I tend to think more of the associations of the shoe – who wears it, is it old-hat, and so on – but I think it's good, although difficult, to keep that fresh attitude. The trainer world is political, but when I see the shoes it all that other stuff seems unimportant and you remember what it's all about.'

puma **brand history**

The history of Puma is a journey through some of the world's greatest sports achievements of the last fifty years or so. Not only that, but trainers with the sign of the leaping cat with the Puma 'Form Stripe' logo have been on the feet of most of the cutting-edge youth movements of each generation during that same time.

The story of Puma and its founder, Rudolph (Rudi) Dassler, began in Germany in 1948 but, as has been discussed previously (*see pages 90–3*), the roots of the company go right back to the 1920s and are inextricably linked with those of adidas, founded by Rudolph's brother Adolph (Adi). However, there is more to Puma than a tale of sibling rivalry. Interestingly, Puma is more

ready than adidas to shed light on the split of the Dassler brothers, but this will be looked at later.

Back in 1924, in more harmonious times, Rudi and Adi Dassler, the sons of a cobbler, formed the company Gebrüder Dassler OHG (Dassler Brothers Ltd) after a period of collaboration on sports shoe development in their hometown of Herzogenaurach, near Nuremberg. 'You cannot play sports wearing shoes that you would walk around town with' were the words of Puma's founder, and it was this sentiment that became the driving force behind the sports shoe improvements that the Dassler brothers introduced.

After initial success and further substantial growth, trouble broke out between

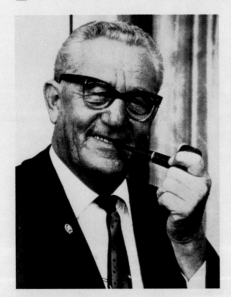

ABOVE One of the Dassler brothers, Puma founder Rudolph Dassler.

LEFT The original Puma logo, complete with the 'leaping cat'.

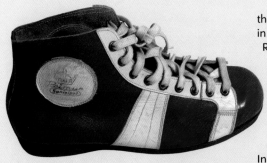

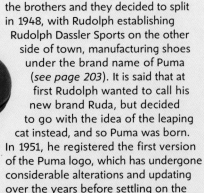

the brothers and they decided to split in 1948, with Rudolph establishing Rudolph Dassler Sports on the other side of town, manufacturing shoes under the brand name of Puma (*see page 203*). It is said that at first Rudolph wanted to call his new brand Ruda, but decided to go with the idea of the leaping cat instead, and so Puma was born. In 1951, he registered the first version of the Puma logo, which has undergone considerable alterations and updating over the years before settling on the incarnation that we are all so familiar with today.

A few years later, in 1958, Puma introduced the now familiar 'Form Stripe', the logo we see on the sides of all Puma shoes to this day. This

addition, however, was not simply an aesthetic design feature; its intention was to provide the shoes with extra strength and durability.

The company went from strength to strength, with Puma-clad runners winning gold medals at various Olympic Games and other international sporting events.

Puma can also lay claim to being the first brand to utilize Velcro straps in 1968, and it was at this time that Puma and adidas were both making inroads into the American market. These German brands went on to dominate the 1970s and their shoes from this era, such as the Clyde and State/Suede, still sell in huge volumes.

It is during these years that Puma achieved the type of cultural following that any manufacturer would die for. Puma was particularly favoured by the brash, new Hip-Hop 'tribe' in the late 1970s/early 1980s (*see pages 20–5*).

ABOVE LEFT Early Super Atoms, featuring Puma's first logo.
LEFT Top Fit, with today's Form Stripe and logo.

In 1986 Puma changed fundamentally, going from a family business to being listed on the German stock exchange, and this corresponded with a general slump in sales for the 'old-skool' brands such as Puma and adidas during the late 1980s and 1990s as new players Nike and Reebok began to enjoy 'their moments in the sun'.

Recently, by combining old designs with new developments, Puma has started to recover market share and is once more becoming one of the major players.

SPORTS STORIES

It's reasonable to say that not every brand of training shoes enjoyed the loyalty or success that has been illustrated by Puma, and the company established particularly successful relationships with soccer superstars such as Pelé of Brazil, Johann Cruyff of Holland and Diego Maradona of Argentina.

Some notable stories are particularly worth the retelling. Johann Cruyff was a sponsored Puma player while, at the same time, his Dutch international team was sponsored by deadly rivals adidas. When Cruyff was playing for his country he would rip off one of the three stripes on his jersey to negate the adidas connection. Such a demonstration would be impossible to imagine with the superstars of today's game.

The world's greatest and most famous soccer player of all time, Pelé, was Puma-clad, and he even developed a range of trainers to go with his endorsement (*see pages 82–4*). Pelé always make a point of tying his shoe laces just before kick-off during the 1970 World Cup to draw attention to his feet for the cameras and the world to see and take note.

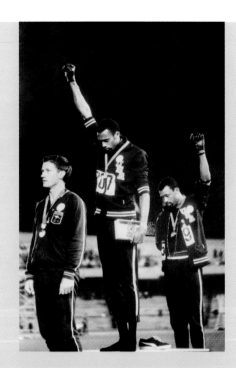

ABOVE Tommy Smith and Jim Hines giving the black power salute in 1968.

In a moment that had enormous cultural significance, American athletes Tommy Smith and Jim Hines gave black-power salutes when receiving their medals at the 1968 Mexico Olympics. Their Puma sneakers were symbolically left on the rostrum and were forever tied to this famous statement.

SIBLING RIVALRY

On either bank of the Aurach River in Bavaria are the headquarters of the two Dassler giants. The extraordinary story of the Dassler family holds all the passion, bitterness and suspense of a real-life soap. 'Dallas on the River Aurach' they call it locally. The personal bitterness that has divided this family for nearly 50 years is equalled only by their ruthless commercial rivalry. According to Puma, the story of the Dassler brothers goes something like this.

Both companies emerged from the genius of Herzogenaurach's village

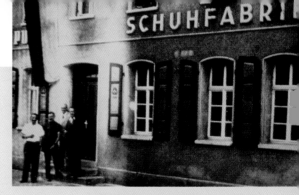

shoemaker, Adi Dassler, and his brother Rudolph. As they struggled to put the business back on its feet after the war their partnership ended in a quarrel so violent that the brothers never spoke to each other for the rest of their lives.

Just how it happened remains a closely guarded secret. Whatever the reason, the result was that Rudolph crossed the river and founded Puma. On the opposite bank, Adi coined the name adidas for his company and so their commercial rivalry began.

Frank Dassler, Rudolph's grandson, stunned family members when he crossed the river and moved into a new home on adidas territory. ' I broke the rules,' says Frank. 'I would hear stories of ... the families refusing to use the same butcher'.

Adi and Rudolph are now both dead, but the rivalry continues to this day.

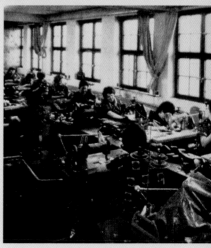

ABOVE RIGHT The original Puma factory in 1948.
RIGHT At the production line inside.

anjan

Based on an original running-shoe profile, this leisure shoe from the 1990s features a lightweight air-mesh upper with an Easy Rider type midsole and outsole. On its release in America the Anjan was a huge success. Its first colourway was green and gold, but since then the shoe has been reissued in various colours.

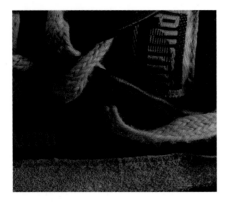

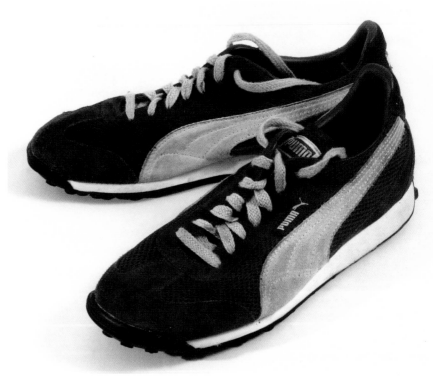

avanti

Puma has recently surged back up the rankings in terms of trainer sales and market share, and models such as the Avanti are at the root of the company's new-found success. Inspired by a running shoe of the 1970s, this modern reworking is aimed squarely at the hugely important fashion and leisure markets.

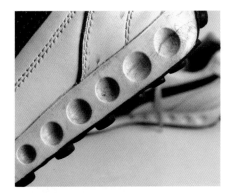

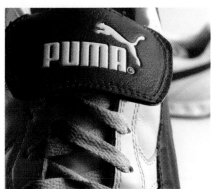

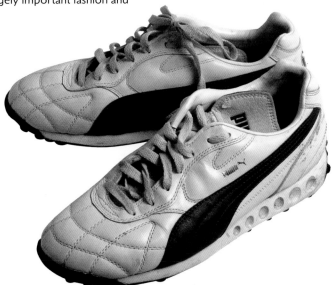

basket

Its as simple as this: the Basket is a leather version of the State/Suede that is a timeless classic on or off the basketball court. The model was available in many style variations, either with a Form Stripe or with perforations, and sometimes as a Super Basket with a better materials specification. All in all, a great shoe.

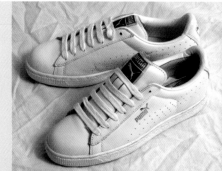

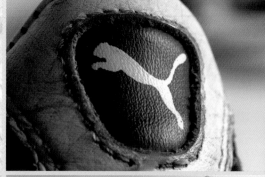

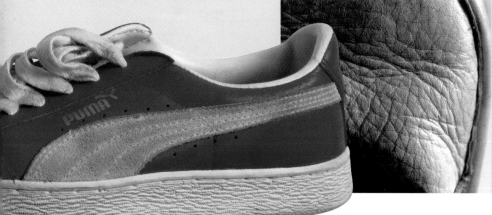

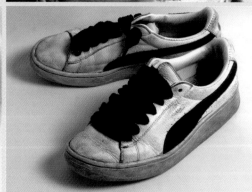

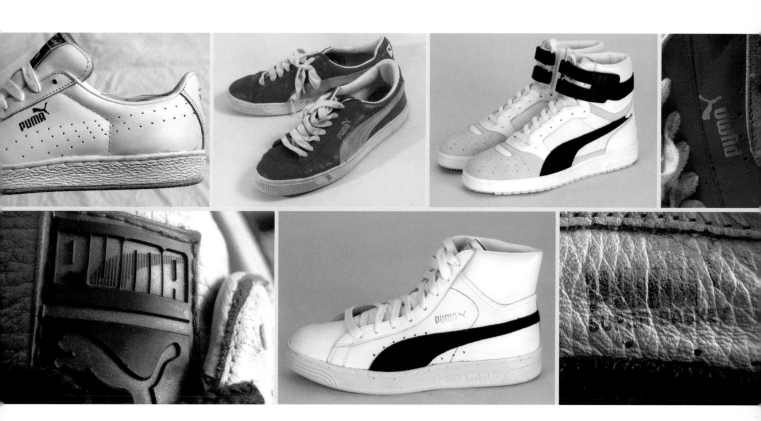

boris becker ace

Here is a classic example of a famous signature shoe. Boris Becker was the youngest male to have won the prestigious Wimbledon Tennis Championships, as well as many other competitions. Puma put the player's signature next to one of their tennis shoe models and so created the soft-leather Boris Becker Ace.

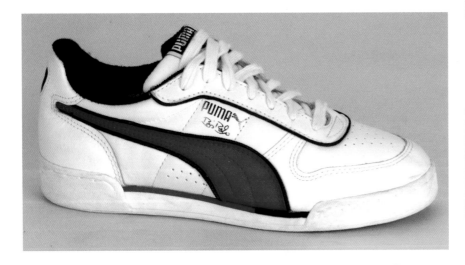

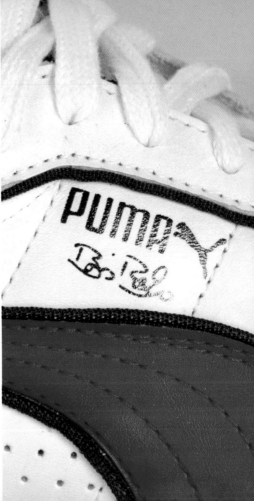

campus hi

This tennis shoe dates from the early 1980s and the hi-top version shown here is extremely rare. With its 'Made In Italy' tag, it is, just as you would expect it to be, a shoe of the highest quality. Take particular note of the lacing system, which features plastic eyelets.

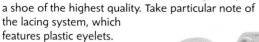

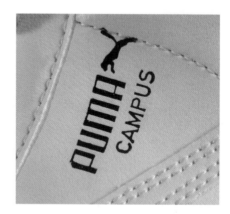

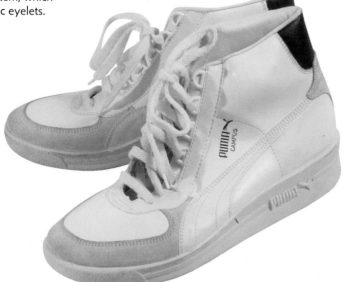

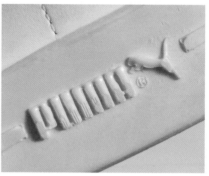

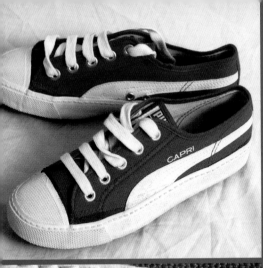

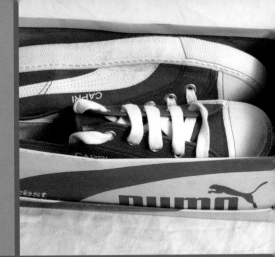

capri

The Capri is an early leisure-shoe release from Puma. This model displays all the hallmarks of the company's first trainers, exhibiting a vulcanized rubber sole and a canvas upper. It was first released in the early 1970s, specifically as a tennis shoe, but it was equally at home on the basketball court.

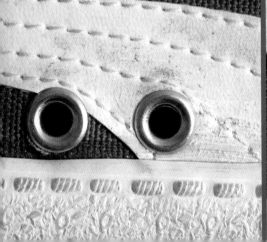

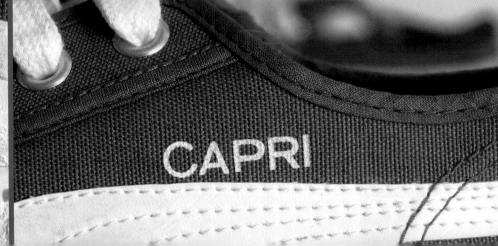

clyde

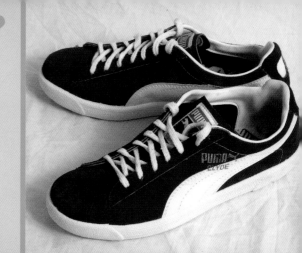

The Clyde is probably one of Puma's most famous and enduringly popular shoes. In fact, it is only a reworked State/Suede, but when they were worn and endorsed by the early 1970s' basketball hero Walt Clyde Frazier, the shoes became incredibly popular and are sought after to this day by collectors.

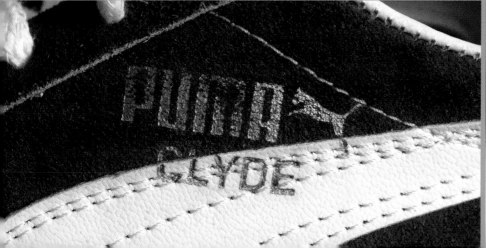

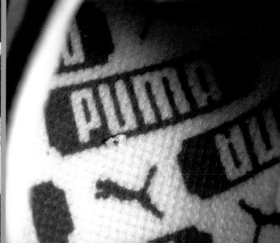

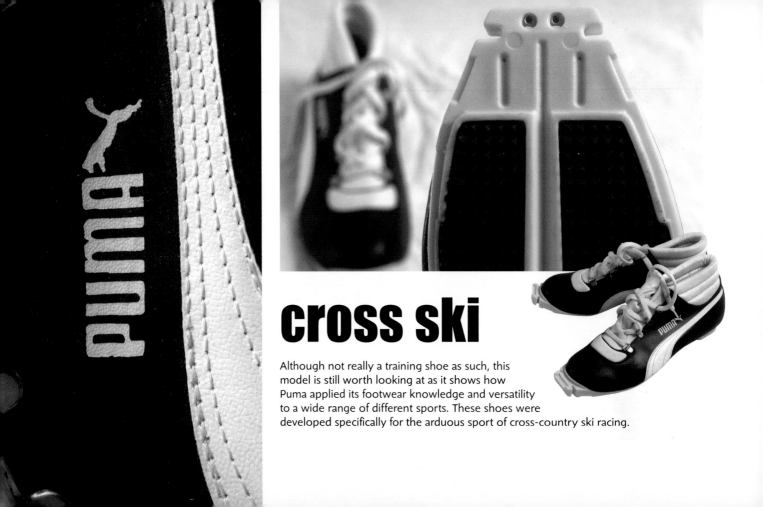

cross ski

Although not really a training shoe as such, this model is still worth looking at as it shows how Puma applied its footwear knowledge and versatility to a wide range of different sports. These shoes were developed specifically for the arduous sport of cross-country ski racing.

easy rider

The Easy Rider model is a hardy perennial and has been around since the early 1970s. It is one of the most famous and popular of trainers from Puma's grand catalogue and was so revolutionary for its time that it caused a real stir on its release. Designed as a jogging and training shoe, with the famous Federbein sole, its silhouette was to be the base of many of Puma's shoes from the same era.

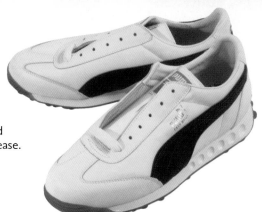

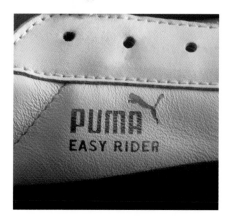

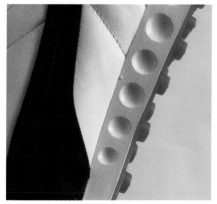

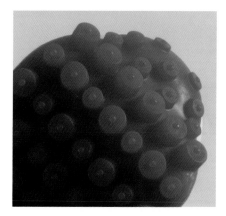

first court super

A ladies tennis shoe first released in the early 1980s, built to last for comfort, performance and superior fit, the First Court Super exhibits the perforation outline of the Form Stripe along the sides, as well as wide velcro straps. The full leather upper features a padded tongue and ankle collar.

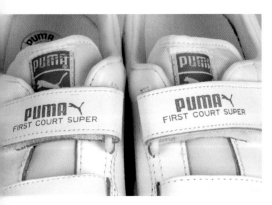

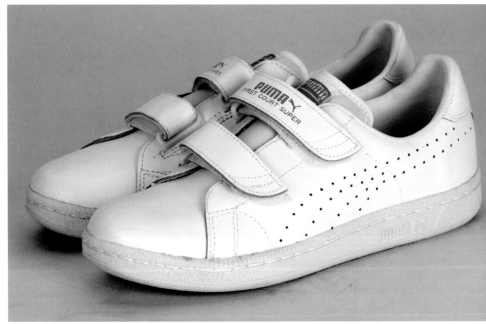

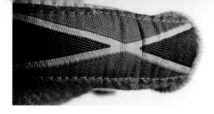

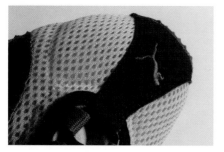

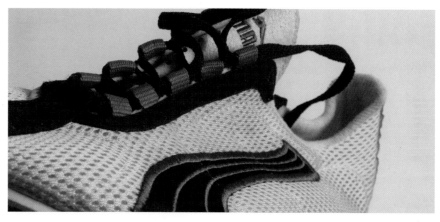

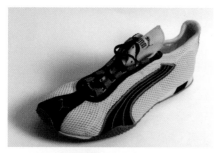

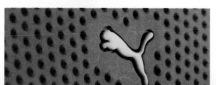

H street

Released in 2003, this shoe is typical of the new trainer aesthetics pushing Puma up the sales charts. The H Street has all the characteristics of a distance track spike, including a low-profile silhouette, minimal outsole and lightweight mesh upper. Here it's in the colours of the Jamaican National and Olympics teams.

jams

This Puma basketball shoe was released in the early 1980s as a late attempt by the company to enter the ever-burgeoning basketball market cornered by adidas, Converse and Nike. It is, arguably, a fact that the reason Puma fell behind in sales terms during the 1980s was that the company did not fully enter this important training-shoe market.

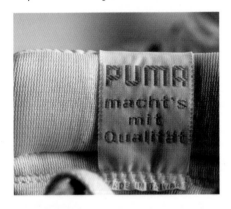

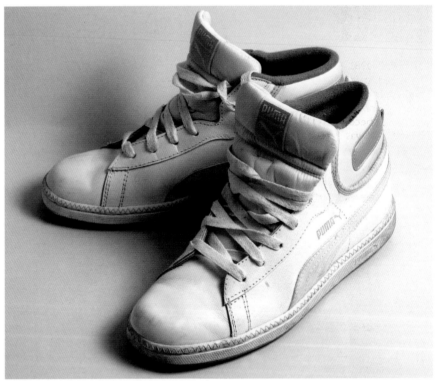

jetter

Released in 1981, the Jetter is a top-quality jogging and racing/running shoe. This superb trainer was designed to withstand approximately 40 miles (65 km) training per week. The shoe's uppers were made from strong Oxford nylon with suede reinforcement panels. The Jetter was made in numerous colourways and went on to become one of the most popular releases from Puma. The Jetter SL (Super Light) was the top of the range of the Jetter series.

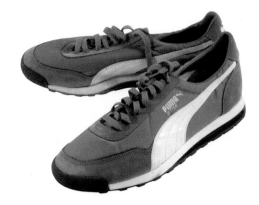

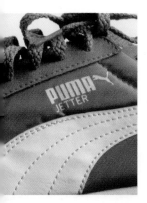

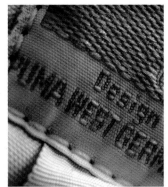

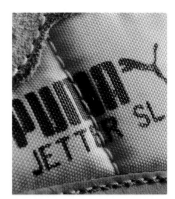

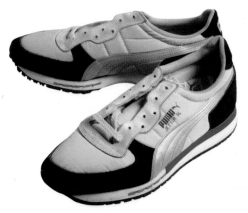

jopper

Unfortunately this wonderful shoe from Puma, released in the 1980s, was made only for children. The Jopper echoed its grown-up brother training shoe, the California, in design but this colourway was unique to the Jopper. A great shame.

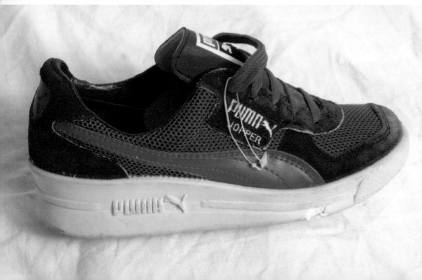

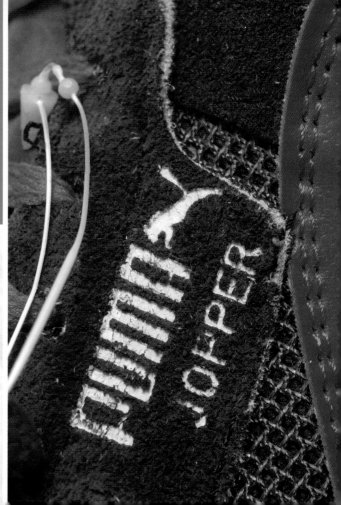

mostro

This recent release is a success story for Puma and has become one of the best-selling modern issues from the brand. The shoes that are helping to propel Puma back up the sales rankings exhibit similar design features to this model. They have the same low- and thin-soled profile as a spiked track-running shoe allied to fashion and comfort, with hard-wearing uppers and straps.

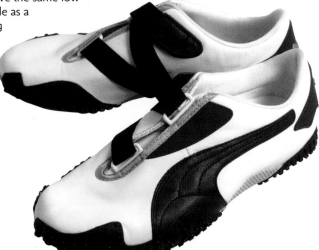

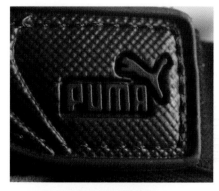

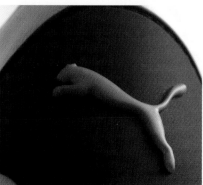

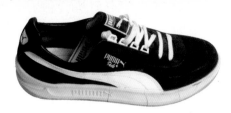
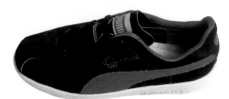
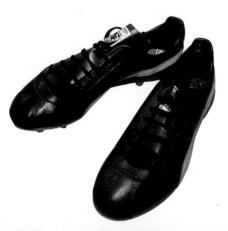
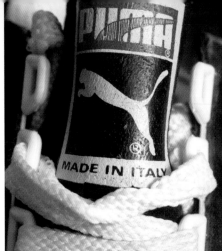

MADE IN ITALY

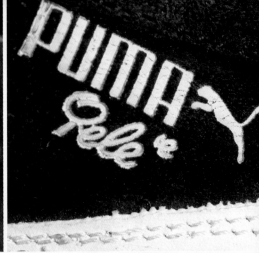

PUMA

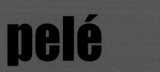

pelé

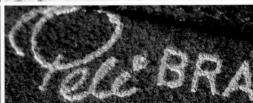

This is arguably the 'holy grail' of signature endorsement shoes for collectors, though not in sales terms. Pelé was probably the best player in the history of the world's most popular sport. Pelé signed to Puma just before the 1970 World Cup, and he continued with a footwear and apparel range for Puma, bringing us the Pelé Brazil, Rio, Grant, Santa and All-Round, to name but a few.

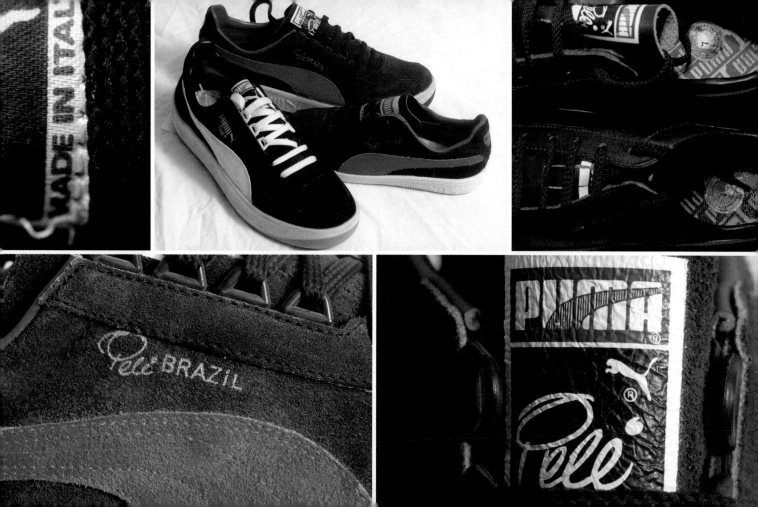

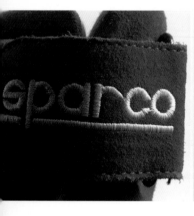

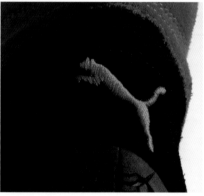

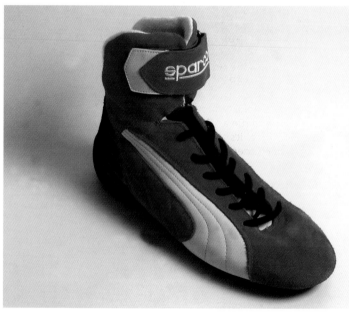

Looking for new markets, the brand turned their expertise to all manner of sporting activities. The Race Cat Hi (also known as the Sparco), was made specifically for motor-racing drivers. This, however, has not stopped it being picked up by a new generation of fashion-orientated buyers.

race cat hi (sparco)

ralph sampson hi

This hi-top shoe was made famous by the legendary Ralph Sampson of the Houston Rockets and his (U.S.) size 17 feet. Ralph said, 'When you play basketball you have to run and you have to last the whole game. It's all in the shoes. Working with Puma's design technicians was good because they knew the technology and I could give them some information about basic support and feelin' good.'

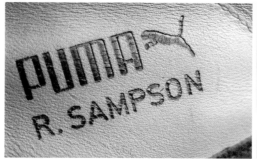

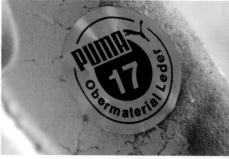

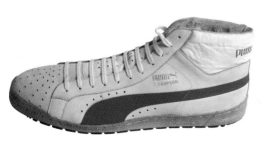

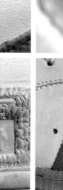

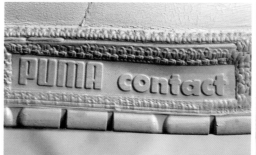

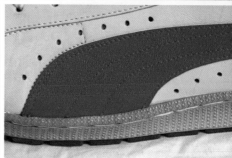

roma

This stand-alone classic training shoe was designed to tie in with the Rome Olympics. It is a 1970s' leather training shoe that is loved and worn by trainer freaks all over the world. The uppers are made of split, bent cowhide and it has a padded tongue and reinforced heel.

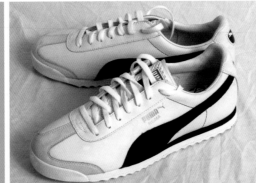

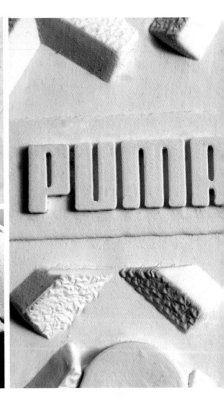

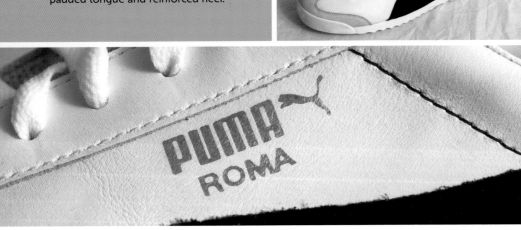

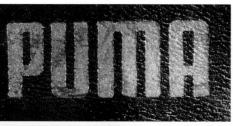

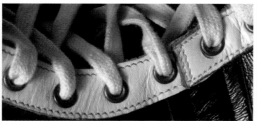

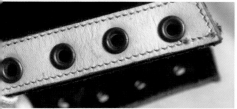

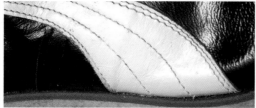

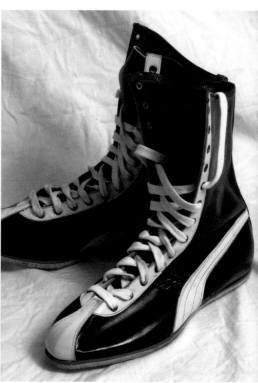

schatten boxing

Boy, these brands made sure they had a presence in every conceivable type of sporting activity. This is a very early Puma and was specifically designed as a boxing shoe. It's doubtful that modern boxers would relish carrying the weight of an all-leather like this around the ring.

sky hi & lo

Introduced in 1982, this is probably
Puma's most successful basketball shoe
ever. Released in hi and lo models for
the prevention of injuries and maximum
comfort, the Sky was worn by many NBA
star teams, including the Boston Celtics.
However, it is more famous for being
adopted and worn by the bboys in the
1980s. This hi-top version is in the L.A.
Lakers colours of purple and yellow.

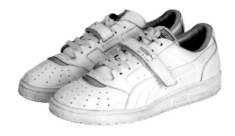

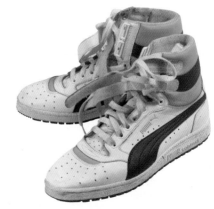

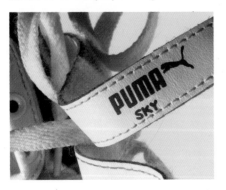

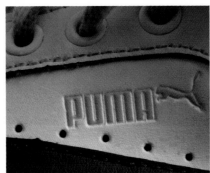

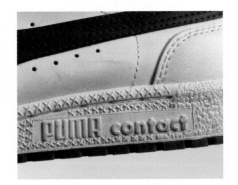

special

You won't see many of these. The Special was developed specifically for wrestling, and was favoured by Japanese Sumo wrestlers. The shoes had a stepped-up heel, which is helpful for wrestling. The leaping cat seen on the back is located in the original 'cat's eyes', which were 'muscle-defined' features, being shaped to fit the achilles tendon.

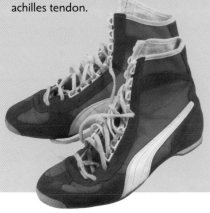

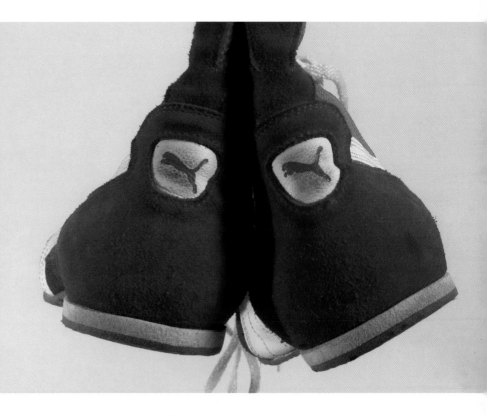

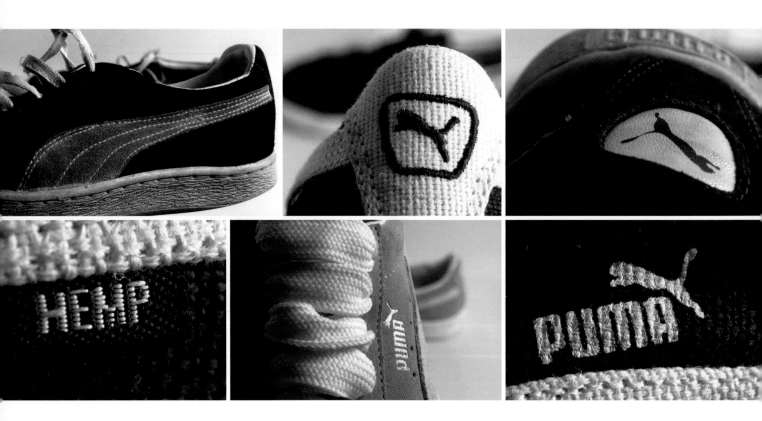

states

Definitely the most well-known and popular of all Puma's shoes, this design classic rightly deserves its place in public affection and in the Hall of Fame (*see pages 52–3*). In the United States, it is marketed as the Suede. The Hemp version (so called because the shoes are made from this material) is sought after and rare.

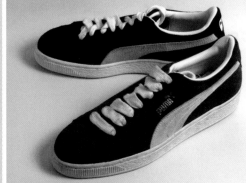

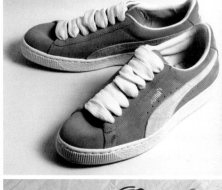

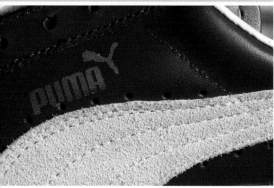

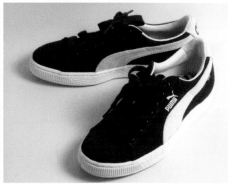

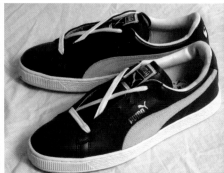

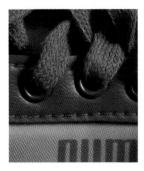
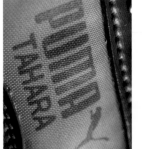
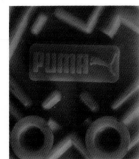

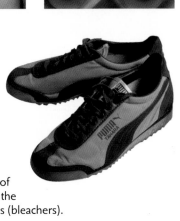

tahara

The Tahara is an indoor training shoe from Puma, featuring a distinctive gum sole and an upper made of a mix of nylon and suede. This shoe is popular with the Casuals and can often be seen on the soccer terraces (bleachers).

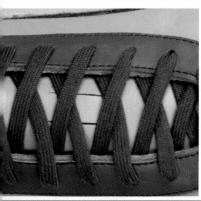

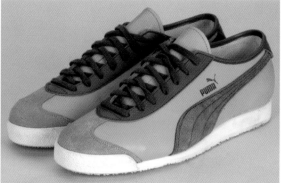

top fit

First introduced in 1963, the Top Fit was designed as an all-round training shoe for athletes preparing to compete in the 1964 Tokyo Olympics. This model was reissued in 2002 for the Japanese market, and only 1,000 pairs were made.

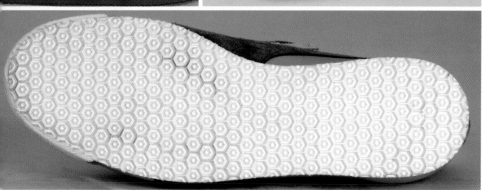

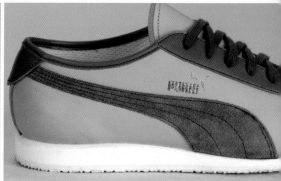

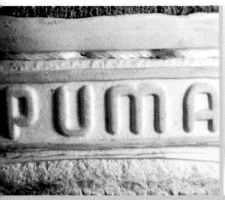

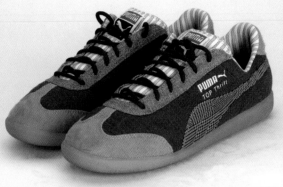

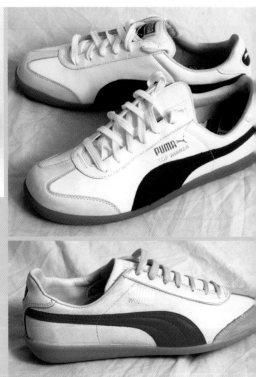

top winner & thrift

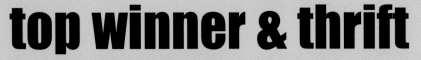

The Winner range was first issued in the 1970s as an indoor training shoe for squash or badminton. The Winner developed, in the 1980s, into the Top Winner and was made from better-quality leather than the initial shoes. The range also spawned the recent release of only 510 pairs of the Top Thrift. This incarnation was a special release and every shoe is uniquely made from second-hand clothing pieces.

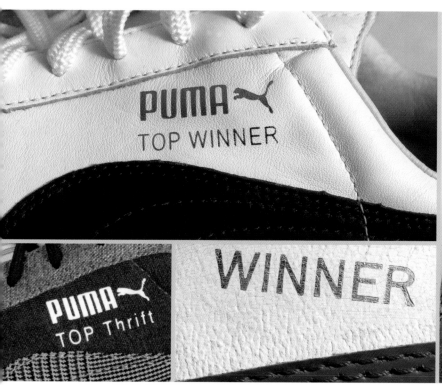

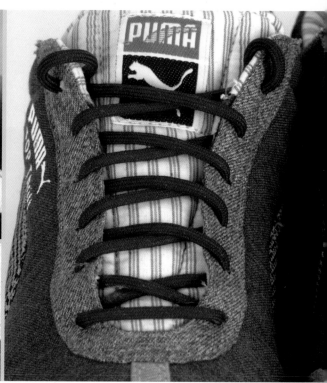

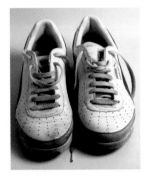
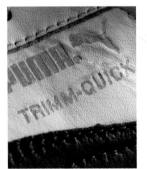
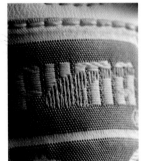

trimm-quick

First released in 1980 as a comfortable training shoe, the Trimm-Quick utilized cowhide uppers, an orthopaedic arch support, and the then new Puma pimple rubber sole. The word 'Trimm' can be roughly translated as 'fitness', and this is exactly what Puma wanted to provide with this shoe.

wimbledon

The Wimbledon, a top-quality tennis shoe, made its debut on the world-famous lawn-tennis court in the 1960s. Before 1988 this shoe was still made in West Germany. The cat branding on the heel has the original cats-eye feature for support. Note, too, how the Form Stripe logo has been outlined in perforations, both for increased air flow and simple good looks.

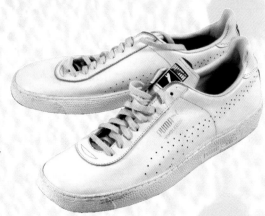

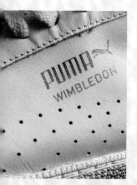 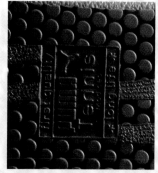 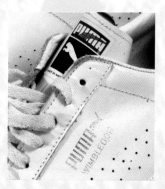 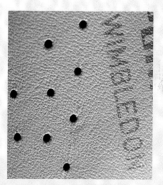 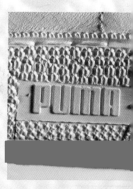

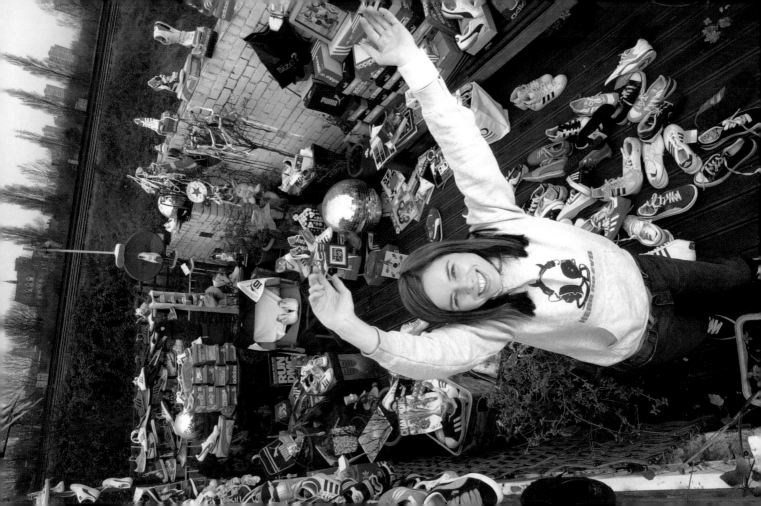

collector
HELEN SWEENEY-DOUGAN

Born in Glasgow, Helen left home at an early age in search of soul music and trainers. Her travels took her across the globe, stopping off in Manchester for Summers of Love '89 and '90. Jumping ship when Acid House turned Ravy Gravy, she headed to New York to see what was going down in Brooklyn. As her trainer collection grew so did her desire to return to London where she is now based.

A true trainer enthusiast, her knowledge, passion and love for the shoes are unbelievable. She has been involved in trainer culture for the last two decades, working as a consultant for many of the top brands while also buying deadstock for her private clients. Many of her shoes feature throughout this book.

NH: Lets start at the beginning, can you remember your first pair?
HSD: I've still got them; they were given to me when I was three months old. They are the cutest, unbranded, soft blue leather with white stripes.

NH: So you've always liked trainers?
HSD: Yeah, I guess so. Trainers were part of growing up, my family all wore them, the boys followed the football in adidas Sambas. My first memory was the boxes. I used to keep my life memories in boxes, a box for each year. I loved the graphics of the Puma cat and adidas

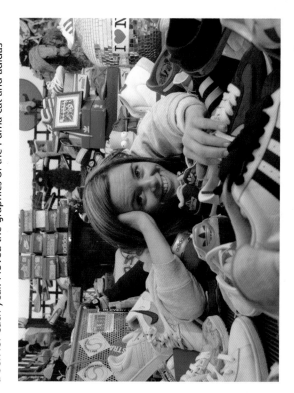

trefoil, I remember tracing these for hours when I was young. Trainers are my life landmarks and to me every shoe holds a memory.

NH: I know that your sisters were a big influence to you.

HSD: They were cool, all into different things. Not crazy on the trainers but they all had them. A fond memory I have was at the height of my sister's punk days (circa 1977), she transformed me into a mini punk – armed with an ink marker and instructions to write 'CRASS' and 'Destroy at random' while I wore my adidas Rom.

NH: Being from the same era as me, did the Casuals influence you in the 1980s?

HSD: Soccer was part of growing up in Glasgow, so soccer culture is something that I was familiar with from an early age. We used to love it when the well-dressed Casuals came to the city; we used to check out their latest footwear, we got a few fashion tips from them. Our hometown crews were not the best styled. I have a lot of shoes that were popular on the terraces (bleachers): the runners, the tennis stars, the city series – many of which I still have.

NH: So you still have shoes from the early days?

HSD: Yes, I have quite a few of them, many rescued from the bin. I have also been able to pick them up cheaply over the years; no one is really interested in U.K. size 4. It's also handy that I am sample size. My shoes hold many memories; I could map out my life with certain ones.

NH: Tell us about a particular pair.

HSD: Okay – Nike Wimbledon bought from my Saturday slave wages in 1983 from Mr Dees in Glasgow. These shoes have been with me on my travels all over the world. If they could talk they would have a few tales. So brief history of the shoe: school, rebellion, soccer games, Acid House, late nights, bad hangovers. Now in need for much tender love and care, dusted down and worn every once in a while.

NH: How many pairs do you have?

HSD: Don't know, maybe about 300 – perhaps more. I've not counted in a long time. I also have a lot of memorabilia, too

NH: You collect all brands?

HSD: Yes, brought up on adidas and Puma. The fact that they are European was important to me. I'm in love with the Dasslers. I got into Nike quite late; I was attracted to the bright colours during the early 1980s. Chuck Ts I have always had a soft spot for. I also like some traditional brands – Bata, Dragon Fly, my Shoalin shoes. If I like the shoe, I buy it, ranging from bargain basement to very expensive.

NH: What about the searching?

HSD: Yes, it's a very important part of it. I have always found it difficult

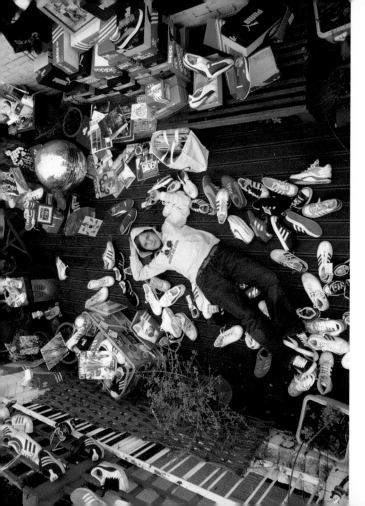

to pass a sports store window. One of the best jobs I have ever had was deadstock sourcing, buying shoes with other people's cash was great. I still do this a little. There is nothing nicer than finding a boxed fresh pair of shoes that have been lying around for years. I've found some great shoes from places that you would least expect. What a hit when you stumble upon a pair and snap them up for next to nothing.

NH: How does it feel being a girl in a world that is male dominated?
HSD: I don't really think about it like that. For me it's fun, I just love the shoes and I am not buying back what I used to have for stupid prices. However, I know how competitive the boys can get, I would not like to be a size 8/9 or be the perfect 10. My male trainer friends love the fact that I am into the shoes. They often stumble across cheap size 4's and buy them for me.

NH: I know it's hard, but who is at your trainer top table?
HSD: I hate questions like this. Currently sitting up front in no particular order are Puma Clydes, signed Run DMC hi tops, Nike Wimbledon, Puma Jam, and adidas Jogger.

NH: What's next?
HSD: My 12-year-old niece has been into trainers for four years and her collection is pretty impressive. For her next birthday we're planning to have a sneaker party and a joint exhibition. She'll also inherit some of my finest shoes. Lucky girl.

reebok **brand history**

This might surprise some people, but Reebok could probably lay rightful claim to being the oldest and most authentic of all trainer brands. Long associated with the birth of aerobics in the 1980s and its well-publicized 'trainer wars' with Nike in the same era, Reebok is regarded as a brash, new upstart – something that could not be further from the truth. Among others, Dunlop lays claim to the earliest sports shoes, and Converse jumps in with Keds. But these brands were primarily producing rubber for various industrial uses, which led on to the development of sports shoes (the earliest examples being the Keds and Chuck Taylors in the Hall of Fame chapter). Reebok, however, began life as a dedicated sports firm making shoes for track athletics.

For the beginning of the Reebok story it's necessary to go back to 1895, to Bolton in England. A local runner with the Bolton Primrose Harriers wanted to develop a pair of running shoes that would improve his performance. This runner was Joseph William

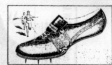

ABOVE A 1936 Foster's advertisement.

Foster. He developed spiked shoes and as word spread, demand grew, and he found himself producing shoes for fellow team members and, later, for those further afield. Foster soon realized he was onto something and turned his hobby into a full-time occupation. The result was Foster Deluxe Spikes.

LEFT Reebok looks to its roots in the 1970s.

In addition to being a budding inventor, it transpired that Foster had yet more strings to his bow. He was quick to realize the potential of advertising and launched a marketing campaign that would have made Phil Knight, the co-founder of Nike, blush. By 1905, Foster was sending out free samples of his shoes to champion runners all over the world. If they replied in glowing terms he would then published their letters of satisfaction in their local countries' press for all to see.

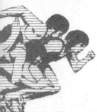

ebok International Ltd., 140–142 Bolton Rd, Bury, BL8 2NP, Gtr. Manchester, England. Tel: 061-761 4965

Joe Foster

Reebok

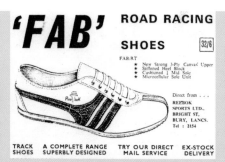

ABOVE A 1958 Reebok advertisement.

However, despite this initial success it was not until 1958 that Foster's grandsons, Joseph and Jeffrey, launched the brand name we are so familiar with today – Reebok. The inspiration for the name of the company came from the fleet-footed African gazelle. The Reebok company eventually absorbed J. W. Foster & Sons, which been established by their entrepreneurial grandfather.

After years of steady but unremarkable growth and development, it was a

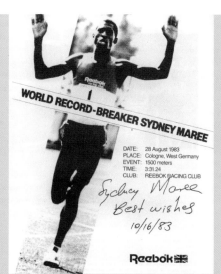

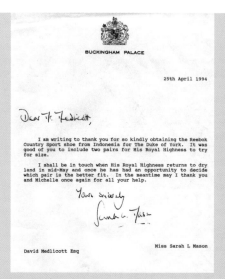

ABOVE LEFT A signed advertisement by record-breaking Sydney Maree.
ABOVE RIGHT Reebok and the Royals.

decision taken by Reebok in the late 1970s that was to make people wake up and remember that the company existed. It seems strange for a company that is arguably the oldest of all the trainer brands to be associated with one of the newest and most 'faddy' of products in the market place today.

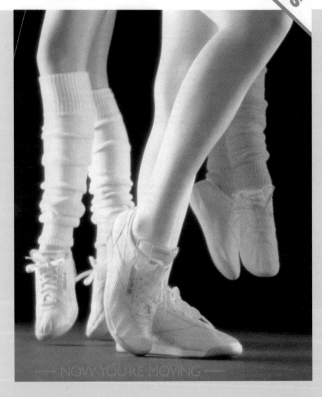

NOW YOU'RE MOVING

Its strategy was simple: even though Reebok's range of sporting goods was being sold in 28 countries worldwide, it was when the company launched in the United States that sales really took off.

In 1979 Reebok gave a distribution licence to Paul Fireman to take the Reebok range to the United States. He introduced three new running shoes and priced them all in excess of $60, making them the most expensive shoes then on the market. It was a risky strategy, but results were spectacular for both Fireman and Reebok. Demand was so overwhelming, with sales of $1.5 million in America alone in 1981, that Reebok's Bolton plant could not keep up with the clamour for its shoes. In order to increase capacity, Reebok took the decision to open a new plant overseas, in South Korea.

This was not all, however, because Reebok – a company perceived as being a brash newcomer – was to change the face of the training-shoe industry for ever. Just when it seemed that trainers were trainers were trainers, Reebok spotted a gap in the market and introduced the Freestyle, a woman's shoe designed specifically for aerobics. The new, primarily female, health and fitness craze took off, and Reebok went along with it. Suddenly, Reebok shot straight to the top of the trainer sales league.

LEFT Reebok pushes the the style, comfort, and fitness craze with this piece of advertising.

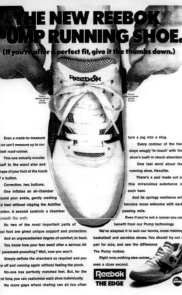

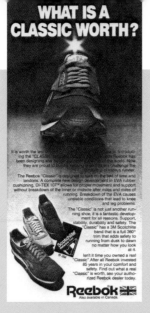

LEFT Two of Reeboks finest – the Pump and Classic Leather.

The 1980s have been described as the era of the 'trainer wars', a battle fought mainly between Reebok and Nike for market dominance and fuelled by enormous advertising budgets. Suddenly, the emphasis was on staying one step ahead by introducing gimmicks. Reebok pulled further away with its Pump Court Victory, forcing Nike to reply with the Air Max. It was at this stage that it seemed that everybody wanted into the market. British Knights appeared on the scene and even L.A. Gear raised its head, going from 1 per cent of market share in 1981 to over 40 per cent three years later (and back down again by the mid 1990s).

However, its association with the trainer fads of the late 1980s came back to haunt Reebok. Unfortunately for Reebok, Nike released the Jordan and, in terms of sales, never looked back. Reebok slipped down the sales charts and, to this day, is trying to shed some of the 'fashion' associations it picked up on its way to the top during this era.

The big brother of the original pump, the Pump Fury, was released in 1990 and was (and, indeed, still is) a huge success for the brand. A technological breakthrough, the shoe was widely acclaimed, but the same features that brought the praise also brought criticism. The shoe was 'loud' and 'futuristic' – the 'gimmick' sneer was applied again.

Today, Reebok is a well-established company, and the Reebok Classic is the biggest-selling shoe in the U.K. Perversely, however, Reebok's name has a greater following worldwide than it has in its own country.

Whatever your thoughts, Reebok has had a major influence on training-shoe development and has a genuine claim to being the oldest of the sneaker brands.

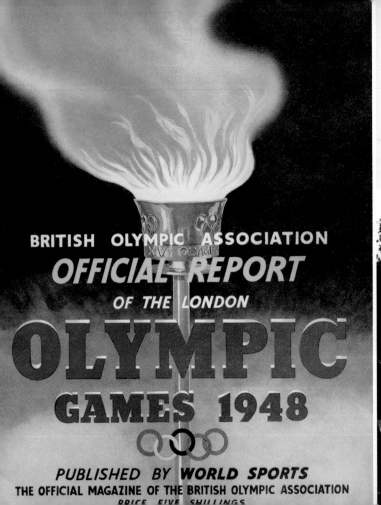

BRITISH OLYMPIC ASSOCIATION
OFFICIAL REPORT
OF THE LONDON
OLYMPIC
GAMES 1948

PUBLISHED BY WORLD SPORTS
THE OFFICIAL MAGAZINE OF THE BRITISH OLYMPIC ASSOCIATION
PRICE FIVE SHILLINGS

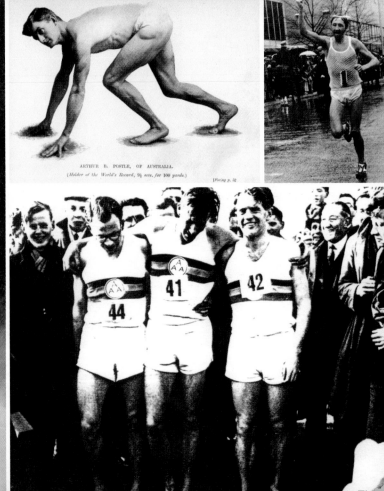

ARTHUR B. POSTLE, OF AUSTRALIA.
(Holder of the World's Record, 9¼ secs. for 100 yards.)

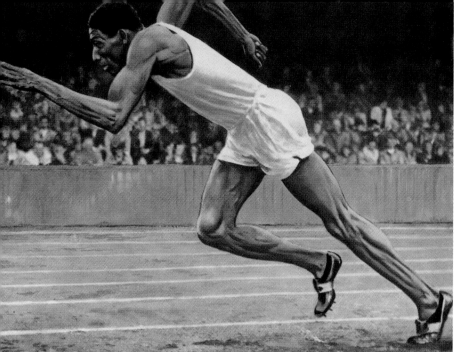

ARTHUR WINT (Jamaica), Olympic 400m. Champion.   Time : 46.2 secs., equals Olympic record.

Mr. J. W. Foster

Death of Well-known Athletics Official

The death, this morning, of Mr. J. W. Foster (52), of 59, Deane-rd., Bolton, will be regretted in athletic circles all over the country and particularly in Bolton and district.

Mr. Foster had been in failing health for five years, and never recovered from a stroke which occurred in October of last year. Deceased founded his successful athletic shoe business at Deane-rd. in 1900, and was well known through this medium abroad as well as at home. The firm of J. W. Foster and Sons manufactures shoes for athletes all over the world, and supplies football training shoes to Association and Rugby football clubs throughout the British Isles, including all the big League clubs.

Mr. J. W. FOSTER

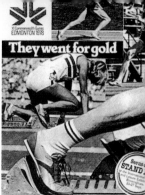

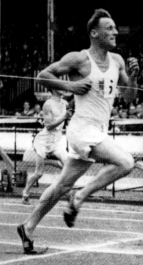

collector

MIKEADELICA

Based in Stockholm, Sweden, Mikeadelica has shot commercials for Ericsson and music videos for such artists as Jay-Jay Johanson and Robyn. He has been collecting sneakers since his teens and used to have one of Sweden's best collections of Reebok Instapumps; unfortunately his storage room was raided by burglars. Here he is interviewed by Johan Wirfalt.

JW: How many sneakers are in your collection?

M: Most of them are in big sacks in the attic, where I probably have around 250 pairs, but I just lost two bags with 40–50 pairs in a burglary and half of them were Reebok Instapump Furys. Now I have only seven pairs left, last week I had 28. I was really devastated, there were a lot of sample-Furys and stuff from L.A. and Hong Kong in those bags.

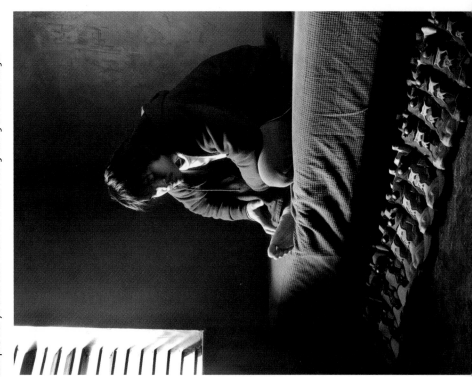

JW: How did you get into collecting?

M: It probably came from breakdancing. I really liked the covers of all the Rocksteady Crew records, the Doze artwork was just amazing. The way he did the sneakers, they looked so damn cool. I got into 'old skool' stuff like adidas Shelltoes and Nike Cortez that way. Later I fell in love with the Reebok Instapump Fury.

JW: So what's the thing with the Fury?

M: The Furys first caught my eye when I was watching an interview with Jackie Chan in the mid 1990s. He was wearing his version, bright yellow and red, and during the interview he was jumping around in the shoes and they looked so comfortable. The Furys were innovative, they glued themselves to your feet and had this bounce when you walked.

JW: How often do you buy new sneakers?

M: I look for new shoes all the time on the internet, and as soon as there's a new Fury colourway that I like, I get it. On average I buy one or two pairs a month, but now I'll have to get more since I was robbed of some of my favourites — I need to buy back the ones I can find. My collecting is built around wearing the shoes, I don't buy anything just to keep it in the box.

I have one pair that luckily wasn't in the bags that were stolen. It's a sample, in black suede with dark burgundy details. They are the only pair I haven't worn yet, I'm afraid I'll mark them.

JW: Which is the most you ever paid for a pair of sneakers?

M: I paid about $US400 for a sample pair of Furys. But usually they come pretty cheap as there aren't too many people collecting them. On the other hand, this makes them harder to find.

JW: Which is your best sneaker find?

M: I found three pairs of boxfresh Furys for U.S. $17 each on a flea market stall in Stockholm. They had belonged to a guy who had moved to the United States, so his mum and dad were just selling all his stuff.

JW: Which are the best sneakers to wear while shooting a video in a steaming hot studio?

M: Reebok Pump Fury, obviously. They're very comfortable. But I'll also have to say Nike Presto, if I don't wear Instapump Furys, I'll go with the Prestos. They sort of fit much the same way.

JW: What are your top five Pump Fury make-ups of all time?

M: Number one spot is the Jackie Chan in bright yellow/red; at number two would be the black suede/dark burgundy; next is the black/grey colourway; then the orange/blue/white; and finally at number five would be the off-white plastic version.

amaze mid

The Amaze Mid was originally a performance basketball shoe released from the late 1980s. Mid-cut and with an ankle strap for extra protection and stability, it was reissued in 2003.

BELOW 'Personalized' for various markets (from left to right): France, Italy, Spain, and Brazil.

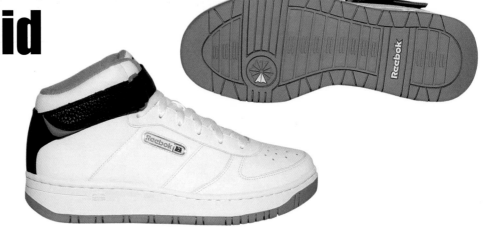

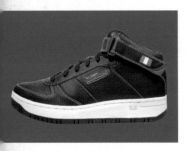
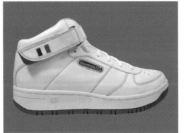
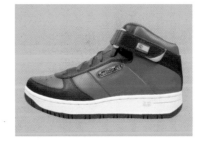
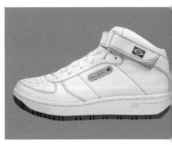

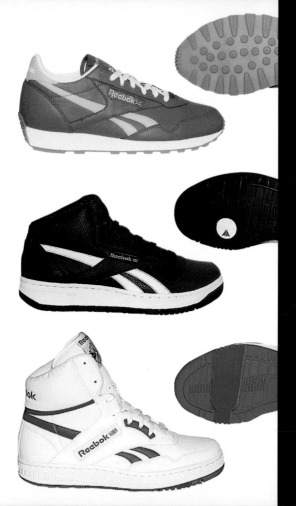

azii

The Azii is one of the original early 1980s' running shoes from Reebok. It was this style of silhouette for which Reebok was renowned before the fitness and basketball booms that made the brand so successful.

bb high post

Reebok made great strides into the American market when it targeted this shoe specifically at the basketball-playing public in the early 1980s. This is the mid-cut model.

bb 4600

From the same era as the High Post, but the Basketball (BB) 4600 was more highly specified in terms of production quality and materials. The high-cut model was designed to give better protection and stability to the ankles.

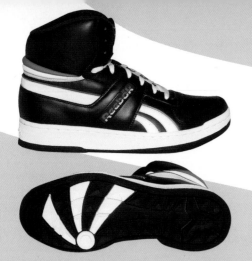

bb 5000

This top-of-the-range basketball shoe from Reebok was issued during the company's decade of growth – the 1980s. In this period, the British firm grew substantially on the back of sales in the basketball market with successful shoes such as the BB 5000.

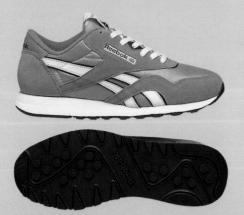

classic nylon

Released as part of Reebok's famous Classic range of shoes, the Classic Nylon was basically the standard running shoe of the 1980s. This was the entry-level model and it was appropriately priced to appeal to the the lower end of the market.

conquest

The Conquest was released at the same time as the Classic Nylon in the 1980s, but it was intended for the more serious runner. The shoe had a higher specification, was made with better-quality materials, such as leather, and was consequently more expensive.

ex o fit

With an eye on developing trends during the 1980s, this rather strange hi-top hybrid shoe was released by Reebok to cater or the new aerobics-mad market. However, it was intended to develop this fitness craze for men.

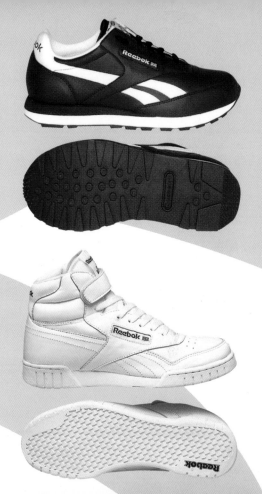

fell runner

This is a late 1970s release from Reebok. The Fell Runner was designed with the brand's Bolton home in England in mind – the shoe was designed for running in the type of upland, cross-country terrain, called 'fells', found around Bolton.

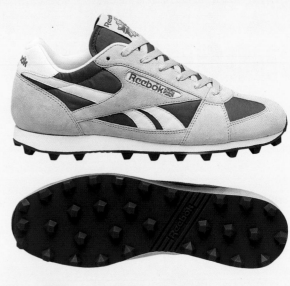

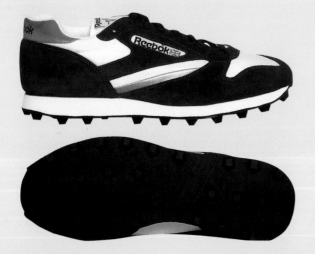

fell racer

The Fell Racer is a lighter version of the Fell Runner and was issued with a generally higher specification. It was a more expensive shoe as a result and was aimed at professional-standard runners.

forza

The Forza is based on a Reebok Classic cycling shoe that was released in the 1970s. This lace-up version was launched in 2002 and is an example of how the brands aim to release shoes for the fashion rather than sporting markets.

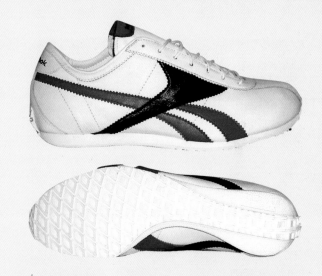

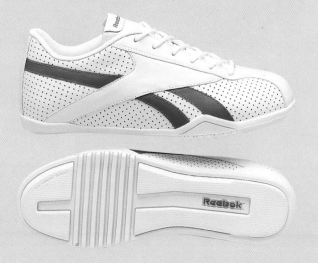

gold medalist

Released in 1984, this was one of the original Reebok track and field shoes. The Gold Medalist was first famously worn by Sergio Bubka at the Barcelona Olympics, and the shoe has been redesigned, recoloured, and re-released.

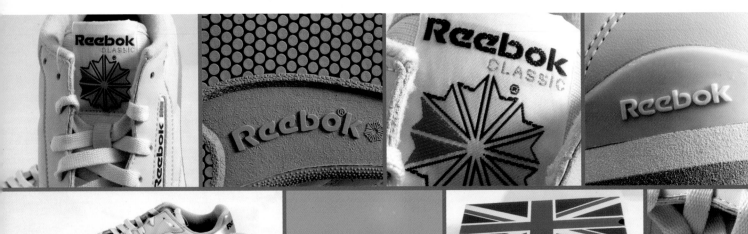

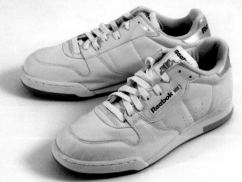

NPC

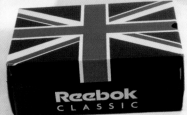

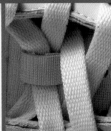

One of the most famous of the Reebok stable, the Newport Classic (or NPC) was released as a soft-leather tennis shoe. However, due to its comfort and classic good looks the NPC became one of the most popular of all Reebok shoes.

phase 1 mesh

The Phase 1 was a model released in the late 1970s. Developed as a road-running shoe, it became popular on the streets of urban U.K. This reissue is made of mesh material with the new fashion market firmly in mind.

PL mid

This is a later development by Reebok for release into the brand's increasingly important basketball market. It is highly specified and features a chunky strap for added protection and comfort.

pro-volley

The Pro-Volley is an example of a sea change in the tennis-shoe market initiated by such players as Andre Agassi and Michael Chang, who ditched the traditional lo-top classic shapes for models that were chunkier and more basketball inspired.

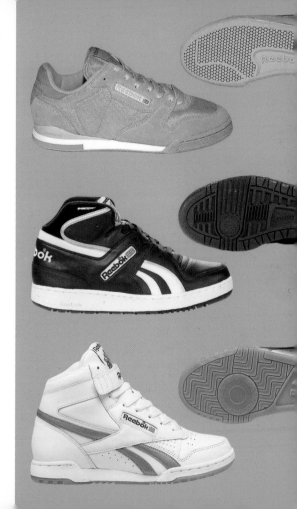

pump front court victory

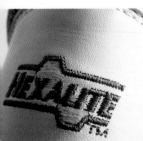

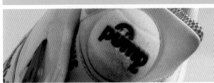

This revolutionary design was released in 1989. The technology allowed you to press or pump the 'basketball' on the tongue to provide an inflatable tongue or bladder for a more secure fit. Not only did it look good, it actually worked.

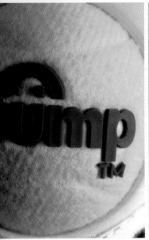

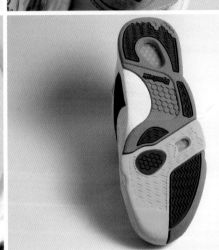

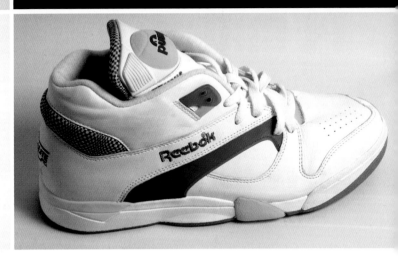

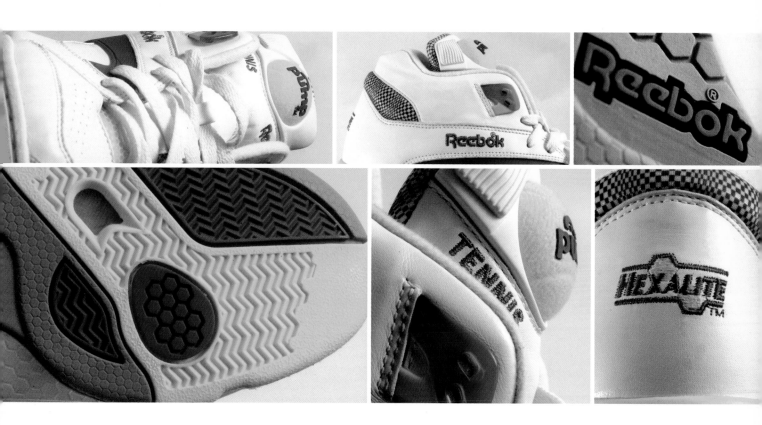

specialist

The Specialist shoe was launched at the end of 2002, and it is based around a running shoe dating from the 1970s. It has been updated, however, with the gum sole wrapping up the side of the shoe. It is available in retro colours in both suedes and leathers.

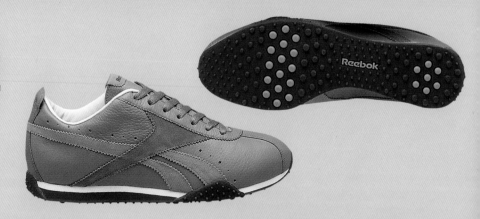

supercourt

Inspired by the indoor court shoes of the 1980s, the original Supercourts were designed for squash, but this model has been revamped. True to the original Reebok styles, the shoe maintains classic design elements, such as side stripes and rotational disks on the sole for stability.

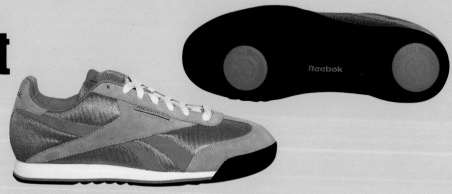

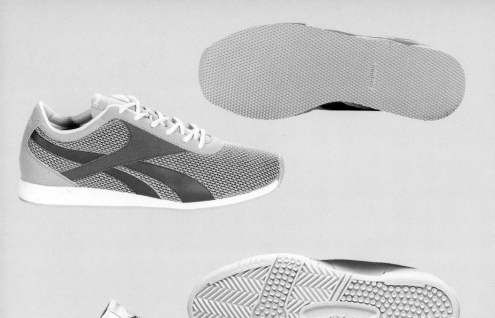

valiant

The Valiant is one of the classic Reebok models reissued in 2003. These new issues employ a range of modern materials and the Valiant is made from a combination of deconstructed mesh and suede. It also features a unique perforated sock liner to provide extra 'breath-a-bility'.

workout

This hugely popular aerobics shoe was released from Reebok in the early 1980s, and it remains a big seller to this day. The Workout was one of the first 'fitness' shoes that was aimed specifically at the male market.

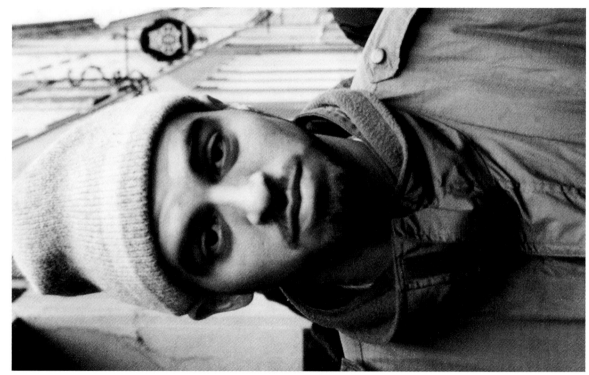

collector
BOBBITO GARCIA

Bobbito (Robert Garcia) is a thirty-three-year-old native New Yorker. Probably the most well-known of all sneaker collectors, Bobbito is well recognized as a sneaker font of knowledge and love Stateside.

'I suppose it was my brother who really got me interested in sneakers, he was a real basketball junky and was really heavily into sneakers. In the 1970s there were real sneaker dudes, people who lived this shit, who lived their stuff. In this era, Hip-Hop was in its pre-pubescent stage, and the sneaker love was coming out of the basketball community. You know, if you play basketball on the streets of New York, then sneakers take a killing, all that concrete. It's important you get a good pair of sneaks, sneaks that last.

It was when Hip-Hop came that sneakers really became seen as status symbols. Those guys kept their shoes shiny white. I was lucky to have been born in an era when I could experience both movements, and they influenced me greatly. I loved Hip-Hop, I wasn't a Hip-Hop head but I dug it and viewed it from the start. I was more a die-hard basketball player, still am. Basketball players really dug their sneakers, and they had a great effect on sneakers themselves. Basketball shoes were made in colours matching the college teams and school colours, so you had all mad sneaker colourways coming out mainly due to basketball. In this way, basketball turned us all on to rare sneakers.

In a way, no one trainer brand dominated, there was no brand loyalty in the early 1970s or 80s. In fact, the scene was kind of anti-brand loyalty. It was all about being one step ahead, if Nike were big, for instance, then I wanted to wear Puma or Avia. It was about being two years ahead of your time.

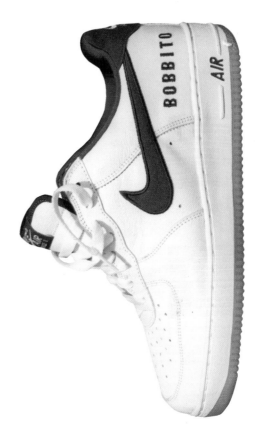

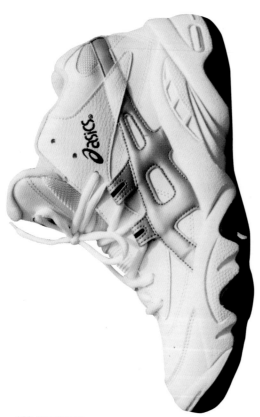

If I had to name my top five sneakers of all time, then in number one place would be Nike Franchise from 1981, in the Columbus colours, light blue/black, and with gummed bottoms. You have to remember, this was the era before Jordan and you just did not see light blue and black sneakers back then.

Nike Air Force 1 released in 1983 is my number two – the pair with the nylon mesh perforation in the toe box. These were the basketball Air Force three years before they were picked up as a fashion shoe. They are really rare. My number three is adidas American from 1975/'76, the basketball shoe.

John Wooden Wilson Bata from 1977 is in number four position. This shoe is in the list because it is so totally rare. In 1977 Bata and Wilson teamed up for some reason to make a sneaker and they made this. It was the first sneaker to use polyurethane and was only out for one year. That sneaker is rare, rare, rare!

And in number five slot is Puma Sky LX from 1986, in the burgundy and white colourway.

I was working with Nike doing consultancy from 1994–97, some paid, some not. The guy I was working with asked me if I designed a shoe what would it be like? I spec'd it and told him that it would be a Nike Air Force 1 Lo with gum-bottom soles and a burgundy suede 'Swoosh' with my name on it. Years later, I met the guy and he gave me the shoes (see page 261). They were just as I'd described. I really didn't think he'd remember me saying all that. But he had. It is a total one off, gum sole and all, the only shoe of its kind in the world. Nice huh?'

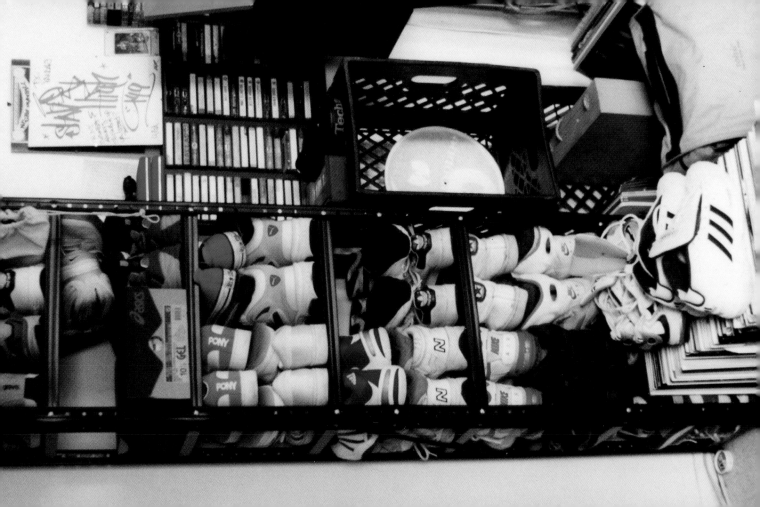

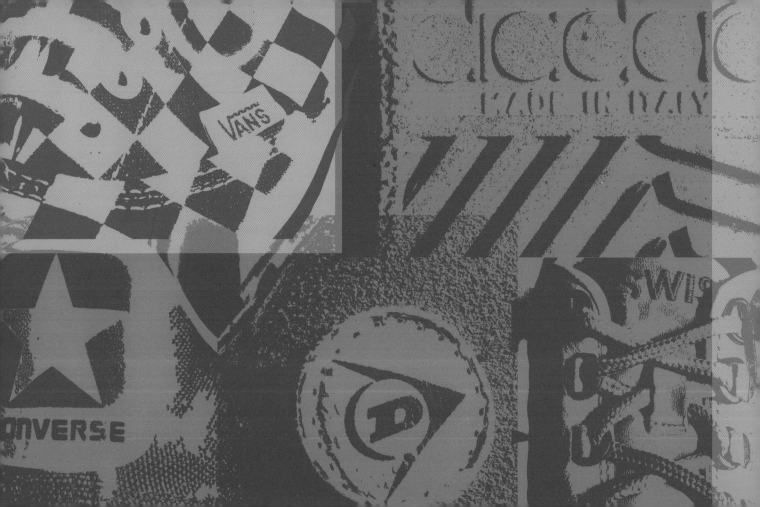

more
players

more players
INTRODUCTION

The splitting up of trainer brands into different categories and chapters is always going to be contentious. It might seem odd to have, for example, Converse or New Balance as entrants in this chapter, as More Players, while some other brands that are far less recognizable today or currently have a smaller share of market sales are assigned to the previous Big Players chapter.

The 'size' of a brand if measured in market sales or consumer loyalty can vary wildly from country to country, even region to region within a country. In addition, market share and loyalties change over time. If we were to draw up a 'big-four' category based on market sales today in the United States, then the list would read: Nike, adidas, Reebok and New Balance. However, if we had compiled the same list even as recently as three years ago, it would have read: Nike, Reebok, Fila and adidas. In between these two times, Asics rose into the mix and then fell back out again, and the same is true of K-Swiss today, which are close to entering the top four. So as you can see, it is not really all that simple to consider any brand a 'major' or 'other player' just in terms of sales at any particular point in time and in one particular country. So, depending on where you are in the world, and when you happen to be reading this book, you will need to apply your own definitions.

Any division of brands needs to take account of such factors as longevity, initial beginnings, product innovation, technological development, history, kudos and so on. Once arrived at, these divisions are not meant to reflect adversely on any brand or model since, as partly touched on in the Hall of Fame, some of the following brands may have contributed hugely to the history of trainers.

Converse was there from the early beginnings and has produced two classics in the Chuck All Star and Jack Purcell that will stand out as trainer icons for all time. New Balance has a long and respected pedigree to rival most in sporting-shoe development. So rather than being a chapter of 'also-rans', this is more a celebration of many fine companies and products (unfortunately there simply is not room for everybody).

This chapter details brands that are large, well-established and respected, as well as those that are lesser known but that have played their part. Sorry if your favourite brand or shoe is missing, but hopefully you will appreciate the wide-ranging feel and eclectic nature of the selection that has been included.

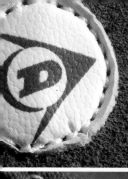
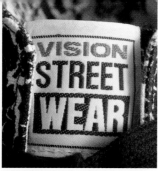
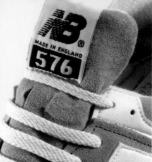
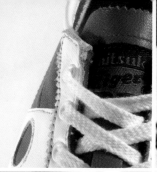
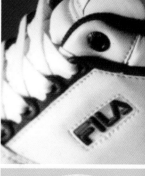

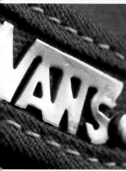
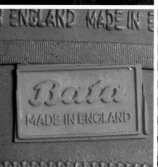
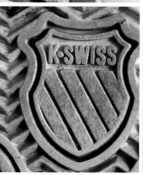
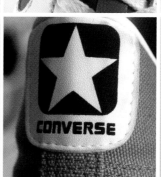
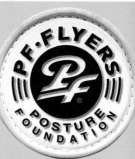

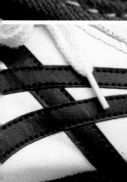
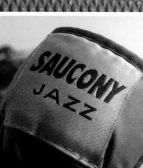
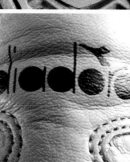
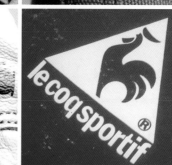
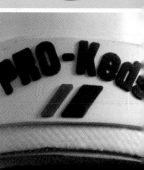

asics/onitsuka tiger brand history

Anima Sana In Corpore Sano
(a sound mind in a sound body)

Taking its name from the initial letters of the Latin phrase above, Asics was founded on the belief that the best way to create a healthy and happy lifestyle is to promote health and fitness. It was in Japan in 1977 that three sports firms – GTO (makers of sportswear and nets), Jelenk (makers of knitwear) and Onitsuka (an established trainer company) – came together to form a new sporting goods company. As successful as Asics is today, the trainer side of the company is firmly rooted in the history of Onitsuka. And the history of Onitsuka is inextricably linked to the passion of one man – Mr Kihachiro Onitsuka.

Onitsuka was particularly affected by the plight of the young delinquents he saw in the towns of recently war-ravaged Japan, and firmly believed that these young people could be rehabilitated through playing sport. It was with this in mind that the company Onitsuka was launched in 1947.

Onitsuka had noted the American enthusiasm for basketball, and it was through this game that he hoped to persuade Japanese kids to participate in sports. Onitsuka was particularly keen to interact with

RIGHT Onitsuka brand creator, Kihachiro Onitsuka.

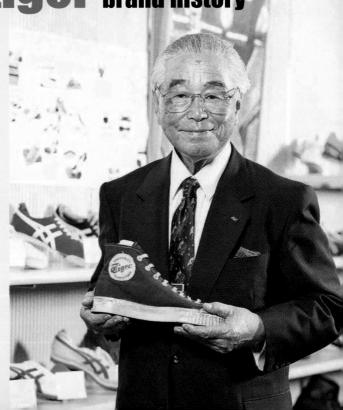

the local basketball sides and frequently consulted with coaches and athletes alike. Often adopting an individual view to the development of his training shoes, one of his technical ideas was for a type of 'sunken sole' (inspired by the gripping ability of an octopus's tentacle) to aid grip on the basketball court. In another example, keen to alleviate the painful affliction of corns forming on runners' feet, Onitsuka's research (inspired by the air-cooling system on a motor bike) led to the Magic Runner. These trainers had improved ventilation to dissipate the heat around the feet that led to the initial inflammation and, hence, to the corns.

Onitsuka went from strength to strength, and in 1957 the company bought the Tiger brand. From this time on, the Tiger logo was used on the sides of their shoes and the company was renamed Onitsuka Tiger. In later years Onitsuka and, today, Asics incorporated the Tiger 'Stripes' on their trainers.

In 1958 Onitsuka celebrated the 10th anniversary of his company in an unusual and enterprising way. He decided that Onitsuka should cease to be a family-run concern and instead become an employee-run business. To achieve this, he distributed 70 percent of company shares to his employees.

In the 1960s Onitsuka become involved with American Phil Knight, the founder of Blue Ribbon Sports, which later evolved into Nike. This story has been told elsewhere in this book, however it is interesting to hear the Japanese slant on the proceedings.

According to Onitsuka, the story is that in the early 1960s a young American, Philip Knight, carried out extensive research on the running-shoe market in the United States and, in 1963, took his results to Japan, where he visited Kihachiro Onitsuka. Philip Knight told the Japanese businessman that he thought his Onitsuka

shoes were the best around and that he would like to market the brand in the United States. Obviously impressed with the American, Onitsuka decided to close the deal with him, whereupon Knight returned home to establish Blue Ribbon Sports Inc. in Oregon.

The Onitsuka-Blue Ribbon partnership proved successful. Then, in 1970, just before Onitsuka could actualize a joint marketing company with Blue Ribbon, Knight made a move that took Onitsuka by surprise – he switched to another manufacturer. Then, when Blue Ribbon sued his company over the use of a sub-brand name, Onitsuka felt even more cheated. Negotiations cost Onitsuka a large amount of money and not much later Blue Ribbon became Nike.

No matter which side of the story you have more sympathy with, the fact is that Asics has played an important role in the history of the training shoe.

magic runner

This is an example of the type of ground-breaking shoes produced by Asics, a company that incorporated the Onitsuka Tiger brand and came into being in 1977. The Magic Runner model was released in 1959 and these shoes were the first worn by champion marathon runner 'barefoot Adebe'. They are an early example of air-cooled shoes, employing holes in the material to allow warm air inside the shoe to escape while drawing in cool air from outside.

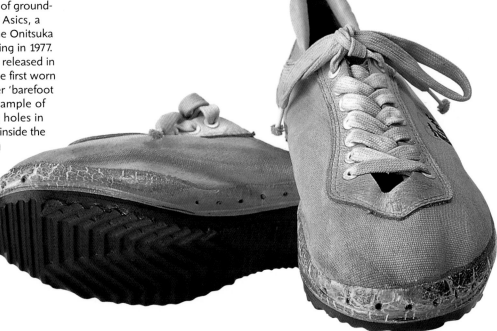

marup nylon

The Marup Nylon was released in 1967 and was a top-of-the-line offering from the long-running and successful Marup series of shoes from Onitsuka. They were designed specifically for marathon and other types of long-distance running. However, due to their colourful and appealing aesthetics, utilizing a nylon upper and a blue instep, these shoes were one of the first of the brand to be picked up by leisure wearers, and 'lesser' athletes. They rapidly became as popular off the track as they were on it.

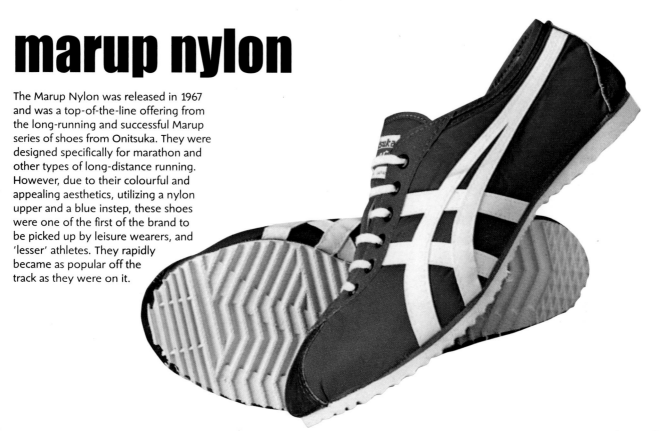

mexico

To introduce Onitsuka Tiger to the wider world, this training shoe was launched in 1966, and it was the first shoe to feature the now famous Tiger 'Stripes'. The sneaker's name comes from the fact that they were worn by the Japanese Olympic team for the 1968 Olympics, held in Mexico. The distinctive stripes were developed to support the midfoot as well as expressing speed, stability, power and safety. The Mexico is available in four colours.

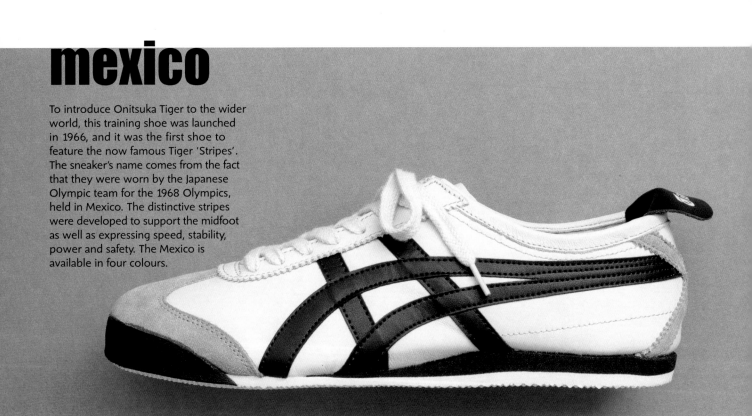

nippon

Although the Nippon series had been around since 1960, it was only when it was especially released as the Nippon 60 for the Japanese Olympic team at the Olympic Games of Rome in 1960 that it gained popularity. The male athletes wore blue shoes, the female athletes red. The Japanese rising sun motif is seen instead of the Tiger 'Stripes' on the upper, and it is supposed to enhance the midfoot.

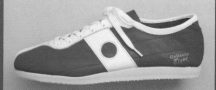

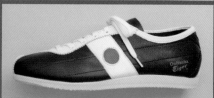

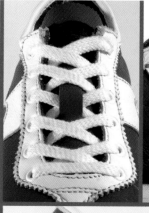

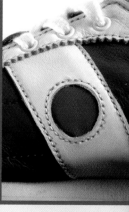

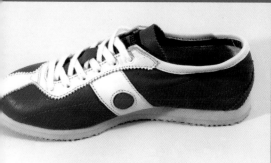

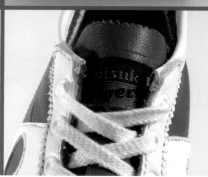

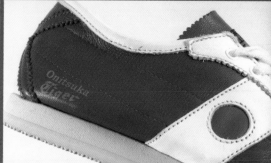

collector
MASAHIRO 'MARK' MINAI

Japan's top collector, Masahiro Minai, rose to fame as the winner of a Japanese quiz show that was literally all about trainers – no mean achievement in his trainer-obsessed country. He is here interviewed by British adidas collector, Robert Brooks.

RB: Introduce yourself and tell us something about your personal trainer history.

MM: My name is Masahiro Minai, but please call me Mark. I'm a freelance journalist mainly writing for fashion and soccer magazines about trainers, sports fashion, soccer shoes and uniforms and so on. I've been doing this since 1998, but before that I worked for Reebok Japan, from 1988 to 1998, as product manager. I was in charge of selecting products, determining price, planning and launching special products for the Japanese market, that type of thing.

RB: What were your first trainers?
MM: My first branded trainers (except for Asics or Onitsuka Tiger) was

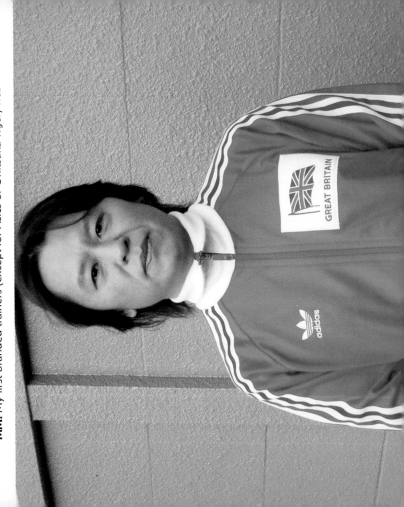

a pair of Nike Leather Cortez DX II in grey/red. I was 15 years old then. After that I purchased Converse All Star Hi in white and black, and then adidas Stan Smiths and K-Swiss.

RB: How many trainers do you think you own now?

MM: Now I must have more than 500 pairs. They are very varied, some old, some the latest models like Nike Shox. I like both high-tech and classic models if they are are good designs and comfortable. For me, the five best trainers are Nike LDV in yellow/blue (made in the U.S.A.); Reebok Pump (the first model); adidas Runner in yellow/blue; Nike Leather Cortez DX II in grey/red (made in Japan); and finally Nike Elite in blue/yellow (made in Japan).

RB: What sneakers are you wearing at the moment?

MM: Right now, adidas Superstar LX with luxury leather uppers and crepe outsoles. These shoes are for any type of fashion style – for example, adidas tracksuits, Levi jeans and even fashion suits. This is the reason I love these shoes.

RB: You have been on television and won a sneaker quiz show in Japan? Tell us about it? What was the competition like?

MM: The show was not really broadcasted recently, it was in 1992. The quiz was on the Fuji TV network, which is one of the most popular networks in Japan, in much the same position as ABC, NBC and CBS are in the United States. The show was very popular and was seen by several million people. Hundreds of people attended the qualifying competition at the TV station, and only the top five scorers got through to appear on television. I was in the United States on business at the time and so couldn't attend the qualifying rounds, but I sent my answers in to the station by fax and my score was number one. So I qualified for the show. The other competitors were a high school student, a famous fashion store clerk, two trainer store clerks and me.

Some of questions were very difficult – for example: 'When Dr. J. was a high school student, he always wore Converse All Star. But what is the one place that he did not wear his Cons?.' The answer is when he went to church.

RB: So how did you prepare for the quiz?

MM: There was nothing to prepare. I just did it!

RB: Did you wear lucky shoes to help get you through the competition?

MM: No, no luck shoes.

RB: What was the prize?

MM: Levi jeans and my travel expenses. The prize was not important. It was the honour of being on the show and winning.

bata brand history

Bata is an apt reminder that trainers are part of a global culture. The business that became the Bata Shoe Organization was established in Zlin, Czechoslovakia, in 1894 by Tomas Bata. Although this business was new, the Bata name had been part of a tradition of shoemaking spanning three hundred years.

By the 1930s Bata had successfully begun making rubber-soled sports and leisure shoes and went on to become the world's leading footwear-exporting company with a unique presence in more than 30 countries.

In 1992, the Organization and family were invited to return to the Czech Republic, where Bata had remained a symbol of national pride and achievement. Today the Bata family continues to be involved, with Thomas G. Bata, the founder's grandson, as chairman.

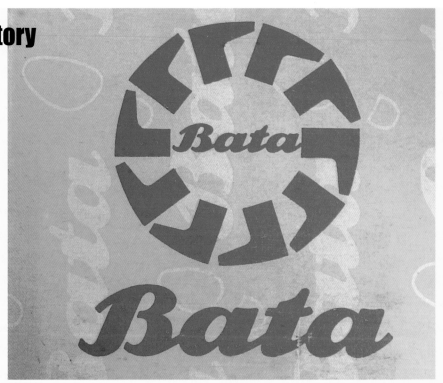

'tennis shoes'

These standard 'tennis shoes' are an offering from the Czech firm Bata and they date from the 1940s. Bata was responsible for setting up its own trading companies in many other countries, establishing itself as the then largest shoe-exporting company in the world. This classic shoe with white canvas uppers on rubber soles was produced by the English trading arm of the Bata Shoe Organization.

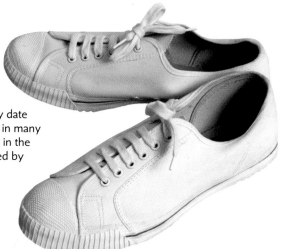

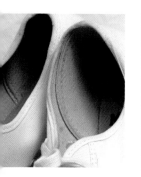
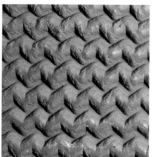
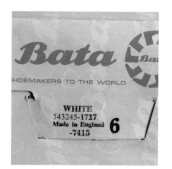
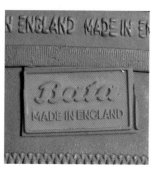
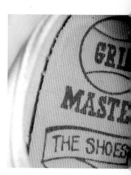

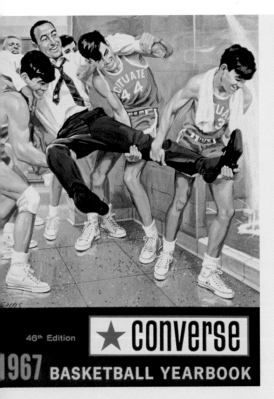

converse brand history

Along with apple pie, Converse and its shoes are as much a part of America as Coca-Cola. On the face of it, it's hard to see why Converse misses The Big Players chapter, but you need to remember that this is a global tale. This is not to say that Converse is not a vitally important company in sneaker history. Its most famous shoes can be seen all over the world, and the All Star (the biggest selling sneaker of all time) and the Jack Purcell were the first sneakers to pass into the leisure and fashion worlds.

The story of this grand old company begins back in 1908 in the State of Massachusetts. It was in this year that the New Hampshire-born Marquis Mills Converse founded the Converse Rubber Shoe Company. Mr Converse was quick to latch onto the potential of the rapidly growing rubber shoe industry after having worked at the local Beacon Falls Rubber Shoe store. Within two years of establishment, Converse had 350 employees producing tough, rubber-soled, protective footwear under brand names including 'Tuff-e-nuff rubbers'. It was at about this time that the company made the fatal mistake of diversifying into other rubber markets, when it branched into making rubber tyres.

Contrary to popular legend, Converse was not the founding father of the sneaker/trainer industry, even though it was involved in its infancy. The Converse company was launched at a time when basketball was, although a minority interest, growing in popularity at an astonishing rate. Basketball players were beginning to utilize rubber-soled leisure or deck shoes, and so Converse diversified away from its main interest in

LEFT Converse yearbook looking earlier than its date.

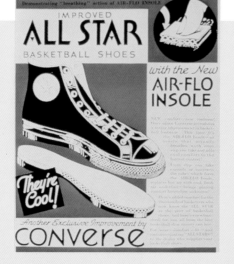

The advertisement text reads:

Cool Comfort for the Hottest Contest — Another Exclusive Improvement in ALL STAR Basketball Shoes — "They BREATHE with every step you take!"

IMPROVED **ALL STAR** BASKETBALL SHOES

with the New **AIR-FLO INSOLE**

They're Cool!

Another Exclusive Improvement by **CONVERSE**

ABOVE An early Converse All Star advertisement.

industrial shoes and began to produce shoes for this relatively new sport.

It was in 1917 that a vital decision was taken when Converse issued a hi-cut shoe designed specifically for basketball. This shoe was intended to maintain productivity in the plant when sales of industrial shoes traditionally fell in the summer. The result was the legendary Converse All Star basketball shoe, which is still sold in a familiar form today.

It was in 1921 that ex-basketball player 'Chuck' Taylor joined the company and began selling the new basketball shoes at classes he held all over the country. Sales boomed, Taylor suggested some additions, such as cushioned heel soles and padding on the ankles, and his signature was added to the shoe – the Chuck Taylor was born. Sales rose again, and Converse as we know the company today became a reality.

However, in these early days Converse was more involved in the tyre market, which proved less than successful. In 1928 the crippling losses of this division took the company into receivership and Marquis Converse left his 'baby'. In 1930, the Stone family became the new owners and stayed in control over the next 40 years, during which time Converse survived and grew by buying many other 'rubber' companies, including tyre and footwear firms such as B.F. Goodrich.

By the 1970s Converse had slipped, falling behind firms such as adidas, who were growing on the back of the running-shoe boom. Converse fought back with semi-successful celebrity endorsements by basketball players like Julius 'Dr J.' Erving, but by the 1980s there had been many plant closures and Converse had become a small part of a larger conglomerate.

However, in 1983 there was a management buy-out and Converse Inc. came into being. Converse has continued its fight back since that time, developing new shoes. But they will forever be associated with their giant twin classics – the All Star and the Jack Purcell.

all star

What can you say about a living legend? It's the biggest selling sneaker of all time, has not really changed in design since its inception in 1916, and is as much a part of popular culture as the sports court? Chucks just seem to go on and on. Seen here in camouflage, this is one of their later design options.

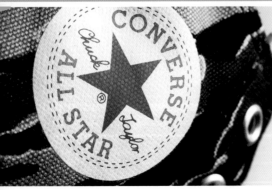

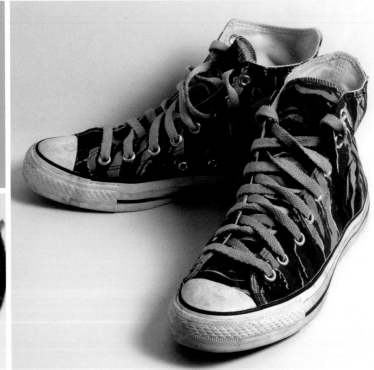

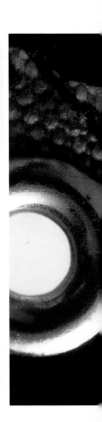

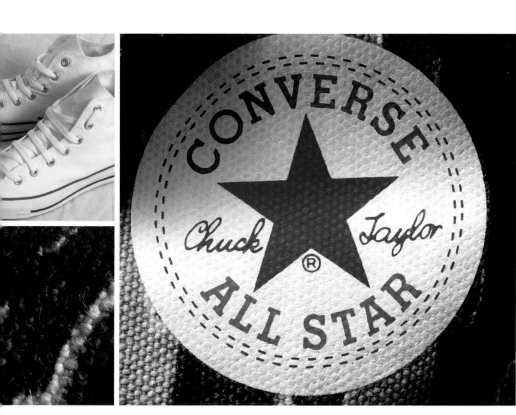

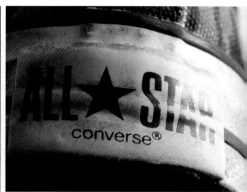

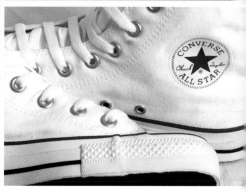

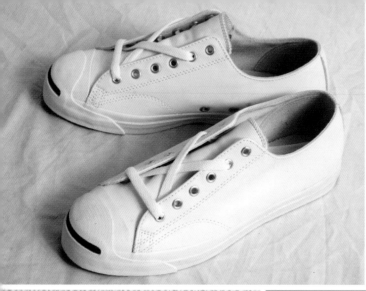

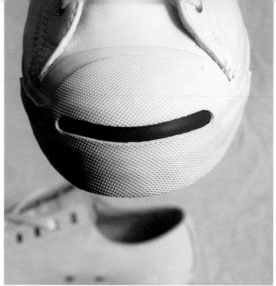

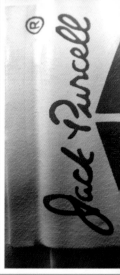

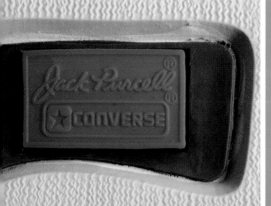

jack purcell

Surprisingly for a shoe that has been adopted as a semi-official leisure footwear item, the Jack Purcell was actually produced by B.F. Goodrich in the 1930s as an indoor court sports shoe. When the famous badminton star of the day, Jack Purcell, added his name to the shoe, a hallowed trainer was born. Converse acquired the rights to make the shoe in the 1970s, since when the model has acquired classic celebrity status.

one star

The One Star is an offering from Converse dating from the mid 1960s. Until the early 1960s the Converse brand had been dominant in the United States. However, with companies such as adidas and Puma entering the market, Converse had to widen the range it offered. The One Star is a lo-cut basketball shoe – the oldest model has a single star, the next oldest two lines, and the most recent issue a star with arrow. When Converse reissued the shoe it was called the Jack Star.

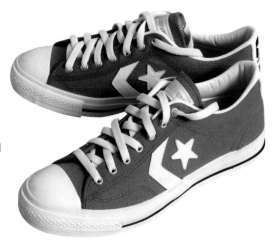

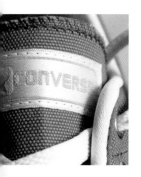 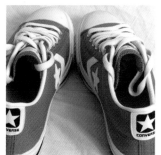 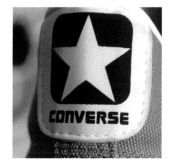 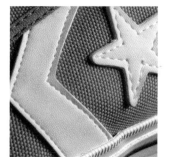 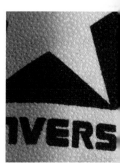

weapon

After years of seeing its market domination eroded by newcomers, Converse made strides to win back some market share. In 1987 the company released the Weapon, a basketball shoe in both hi and lo versions and myriad colours to match those of the NBA teams. This model is the most famous Magic Johnson colourway.

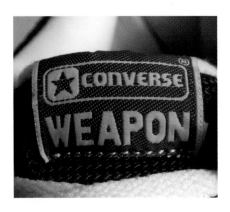

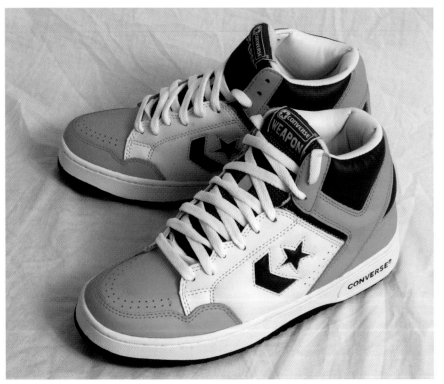

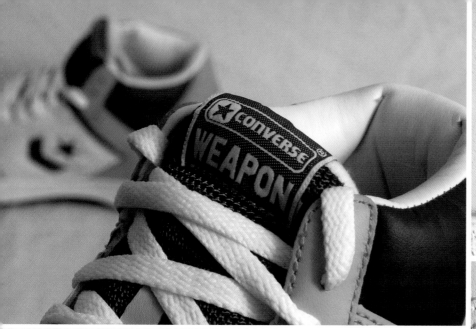

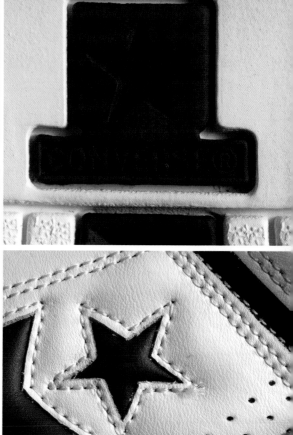

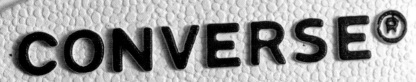

diadora **brand history**

You have got to hand it to the Italians. Whatever they do, they do it with style. Always fashion- and sports-obsessed, Diadora, along with fellow Italian company Fila, are the established Italian contributors to trainer design.

Marcello Danielli established Diadora in a post-war-ravaged Italy in 1948. Although best known as being based in Treviso, the company's earliest beginnings are in the tiny north Italian town of Cerano San Marco. It was from this base that Diadora took its first steps into the sporting world, initially designing all forms of sporting equipment. To this day, the company is still more involved in football and tennis, and its shoes reflect these influences.

Diadora is known in the U.K. largely because of a single pair of shoes – the Borg Elite – which achieved legendary status among the soccer-following culture of Britain. The brand also had shoes endorsed by such luminaries as Boris Becker and Ed Moses. The Ed Moses trainers are super-rare and I would love to add them to my collection.

In 1998 Diadora were acquired by Invicta, the number one sports-utility firm in Italy, whose backpacks are seen on touring Italian kids the world over. With this new backing, Diadora is looking heavily to its heritage and is reissuing such favourites as the Elite, Rally and Equipe.

RIGHT This Diadora advertisement milks its 'Casual heritage'.

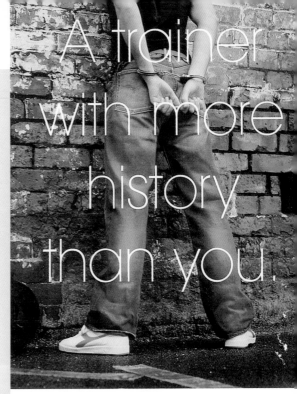

A trainer with more history than you.

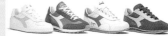

Available at Aspecto, Office, Schuh, Size and Sole Trader.

elite

The Elite was issued in the late 1970s. Although designed as a tennis shoe, and with uppers made of the finest kangaroo leather, it became massively popular with the Casuals in the U.K. It became the Borg Elite when the legendary tennis player added his endorsement to the model in 1978. It was in these shoes that he won five Wimbledon championships.

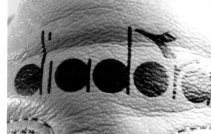

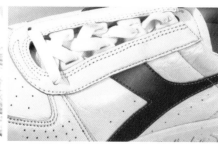

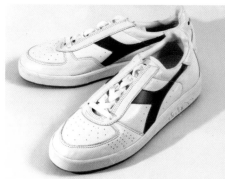

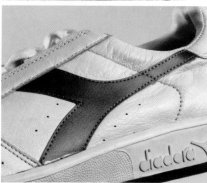

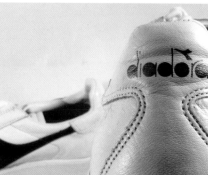

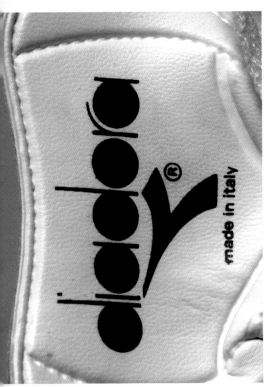

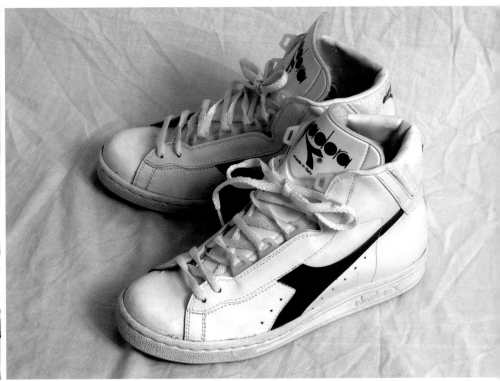

sky high

This basketball shoe is a rare offering from Diadora. It's not surprising that soccer-mad Italy did not have too much to do with basketball, but Diadora, along with others makers in Europe, woke up to the growing popularity of basketball shoes and produced the Sky High as a move away from their traditional markets of soccer and tennis footwear.

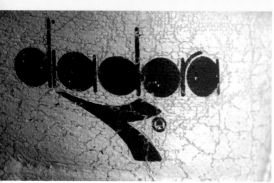

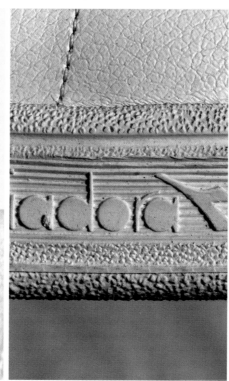

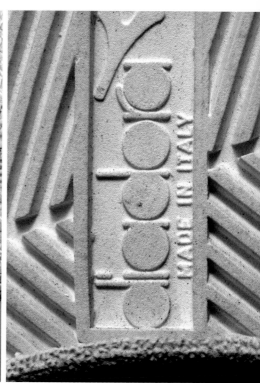

dunlop brand history

Fighting the good fight along with its British compatriot Reebok, Dunlop can lay claim to the earliest forays into trainer development against trans-Atlantic opposition led by Converse. It was in Liverpool in 1830 that John Boyd Dunlop founded the Liverpool Rubber Company, and it was Mr Dunlop who discovered how to bond canvas to rubber, utilizing this new technique in a variety of processes including tyre production. However, of a little more interest to us is Dunlop's application of his process to making an early form of 'plimsolls'. These shoes, although worn by rich Victorians at the beach, were not quite sports shoes. If their main use had been for sports, then Dunlop definitely would be the number one entry in our Hall of Fame.

However, it was not until 1928 that the Dunlop Sports Company was formed. Though the plimsolls might have been worn for sport prior to this date, they do not quite compete with the specialist basketball shoes, the All Stars, made by Converse in 1917.

In any event, Dunlop can certainly trace its sporting heritage back to the very early days. Dunlop sports shoes are mainly known for the famous Green Flash, which was produced in 1933 and worn by British tennis legend Fred Perry on his way to three Wimbledon titles. However, Dunlop does have more strings to its bow. The Green Flash came in different specifications and colourways, such as the amber, blue, gold and silver flash, as well as a pink model 'for the ladies'.

RIGHT Advertisement for the Dunlop Green Flash tennis shoes, a model that first went into production in 1933.

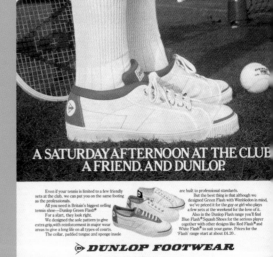

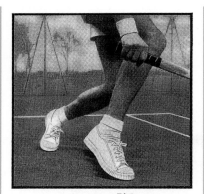

You get *more life* out of
DUNLOP FOOTWEAR

GAME . . . SET . . . MATCH . . . Dunlop
Speciality Sports Shoes give you the professional footgrip you need. They are
specially constructed to stand the strain of
fast tennis on hard or grass courts alike.
Take the GREEN FLASH for example, it has a
soft sponge padded tongue to stop chafing,

ventilating eyelets for foot comfort, the
Dunlop green moulded sole with herringbone pattern, rot-resistant canvas lining and
sponge arch support. It's the choice of
champions. Boys', Women's and Men's
sizes from 29/9d. to 33/11d. Also available
with the special black hard court sole.

BLUE FLASH. Top sportsman sure says in this shoe, volley their way to victory on hard or grass courts. With its rot-resistant lining specially constructed to avoid chafing, and its sponge arch-support in-sole for maximum comfort, this shoe is a winner! Boys', Women's and Men's (in half sizes) from 22/9d.

RED FLASH. Thissmart Oxfordstyleshoe is the sportsman's favourite everywhere and specially priced to suit everyone's pocket. Has soft sponge insole and tough duck crepe sole. Boys', Women's and Men's from 14/11d. Also available in hard-to-wear style—Boys', Women's and Men's from 23/11d.

VENTROL. Here's the family man's sports shoe, fit for any game from a toddler's test match to a fast game of squash. In White canvas with strong duck crepe pattern sole. All family sizes from 7/11d. Also **TENSY—**a sturdy Oxford that's just right for the P.T. enthusiast. Constructed to stand loss of hard wear. Dark crepe sole. In Black or Tan. All sizes from 7/11d.

ABOVE This advertisement from the 1950s reveals Dunlop's self-image.

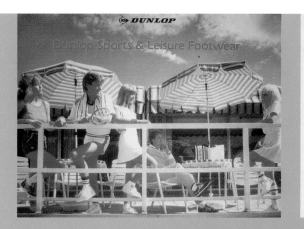

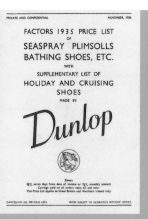

ABOVE A 1970s' feel for Dunlop contrasted with its 1930s heritage.

With such a background it seems strange that Dunlop has drifted along while other brands have grown. Perhaps an anecdote about the Dunlop board in the early 1970s points to the problem. During her illustrious reign as international tennis champion, Steffi Graf went on record as saying that she thought that her Dunlop racket was so good she would use it for free, never mind being paid for the sports endorsements. On hearing of this free publicity and promotion of its product, the response from the Dunlop board was not to contact Miss Graf to thanks her or to make use of this publicity coup. Instead, a call was made to the German superstar endeavouring to take her up on her generous offer.

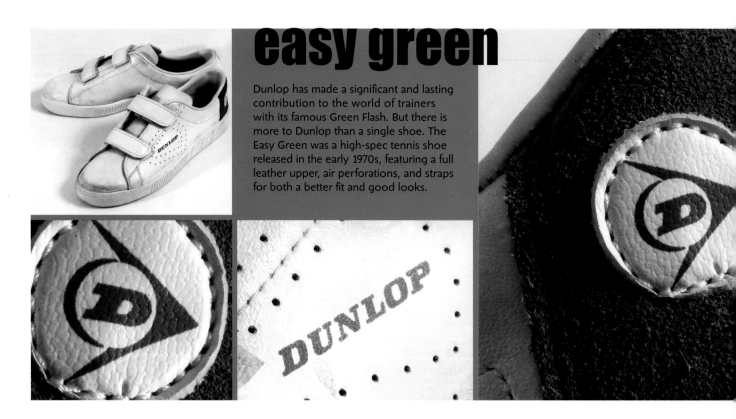

easy green

Dunlop has made a significant and lasting contribution to the world of trainers with its famous Green Flash. But there is more to Dunlop than a single shoe. The Easy Green was a high-spec tennis shoe released in the early 1970s, featuring a full leather upper, air perforations, and straps for both a better fit and good looks.

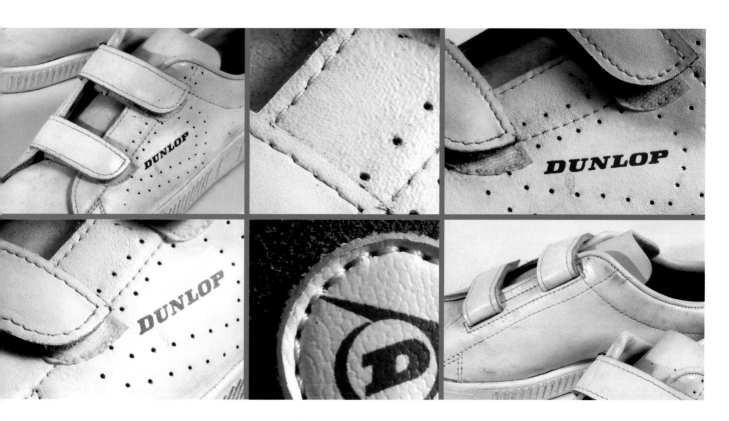

fila brand history

Fila was established in 1911 in Italy as a textiles company making underwear, and it entered the sporting world only in 1973. The red of Fila's badge expresses sunshine and the blue the Mediterranean sea.

It was tennis that provided Fila with entry into the big-time sporting world, especially with Bjorn Borg winning Wimbledon five times wearing their clothes. However, Fila's serious presence in the trainer world dates only from the mid 1980s. In the United States its focus was on basketball shoes, while in the U.K. it concentrated on producing Reebok look-a-likes.

RIGHT Fitness Hiker.

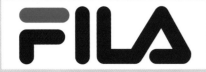

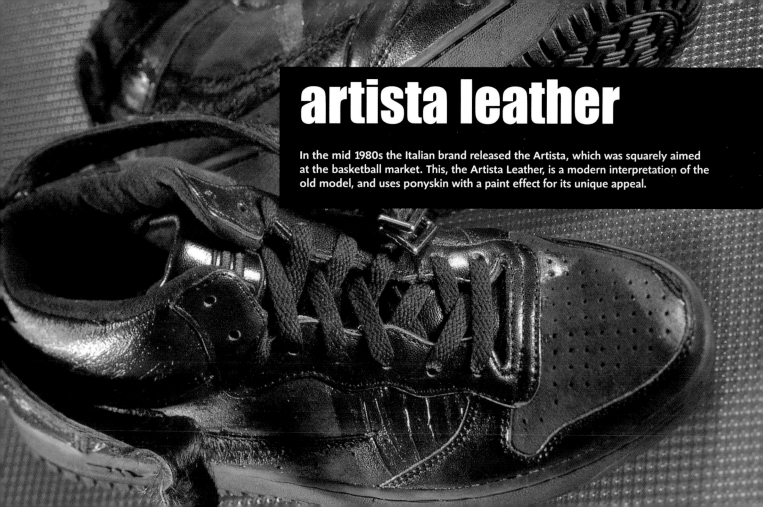

artista leather

In the mid 1980s the Italian brand released the Artista, which was squarely aimed at the basketball market. This, the Artista Leather, is a modern interpretation of the old model, and uses ponyskin with a paint effect for its unique appeal.

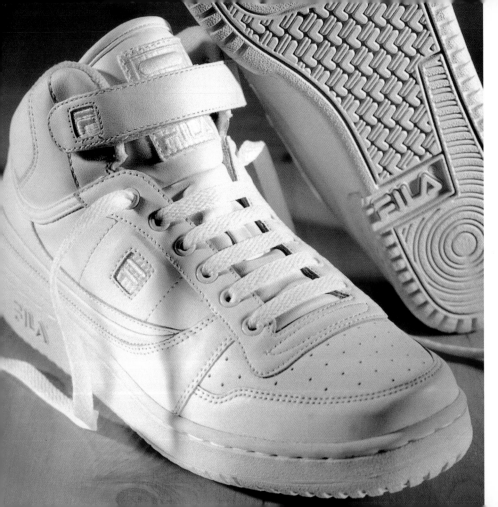

bb 84 mid

An example of Fila's successful forays into the American basketball shoe market, the BB 84 Mid was released in the late 1980s as a mid-cut basketball boot utilizing a Velcro cross-strap. It was reissued in 2003 on the back of a 1980s' revival. Surprisingly, Fila has always been bigger in the United States than in Europe.

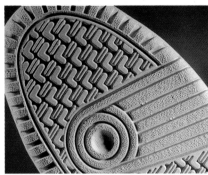

real targa

This model, the Real Targa, was released specifically for the tennis market – an area in which Fila excelled. This model came out toward the end of the 1980s and features a rubberized Fila logo.

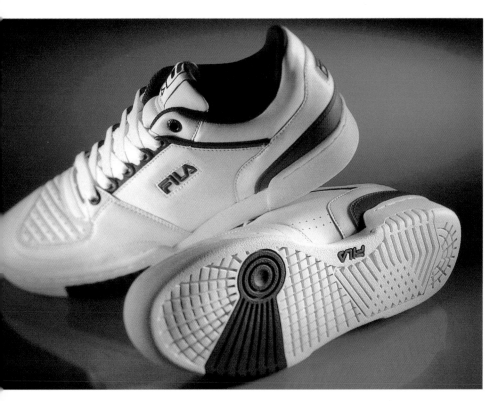

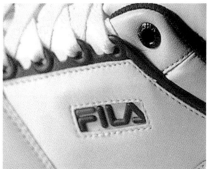

K-SWISS brand history

Although K-Swiss is best known for its connection with tennis, the company was, in fact, inspired by mountain climbing. It was in 1966 that two Swiss brothers set up the company in their adopted home of California, America. Not happy with the tennis shoes then available, the brothers decided to create trainers with the strength and comfort they knew from wearing mountain-climbing shoes.

K-Swiss has grown steadily, but is really famous only for its K-Swiss Classic tennis shoe, whose design has not much altered over the years. The characteristic five stripes on the shoe's side are intended to prevent the upper leather from stretching. The shoes are also noted for utilizing just three pieces of leather. These are tanned twice and then stitched together to help give the comfort with which K-Swiss is associated.

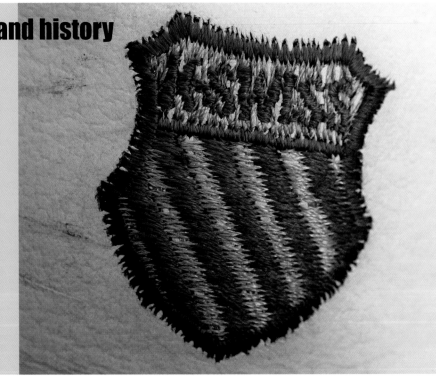

classic

The Classic is so synonymous with K-Swiss that people often think it is the name of the brand. Released as a highly specified tennis shoe in 1966 it became instantly popular, due largely to its innovative production techniques and the quality of the finish. It uses smooth, full-grain leather uppers and exhibits all of K-Swiss signatures: three-piece toe, the five stripes and D-rings for the laces.

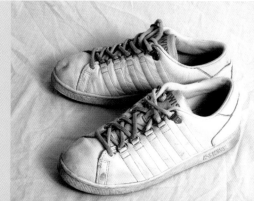
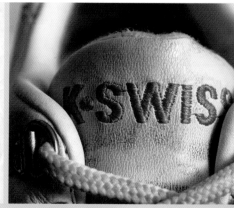
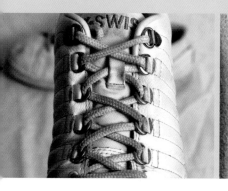
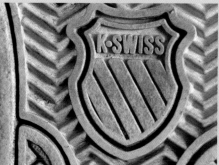
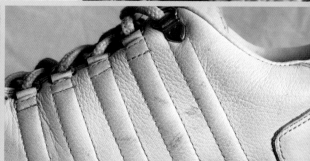

le coq sportif brand history

The Le Coq Sportif story has its roots in the early 1900s in France with Emile Camuset, a manufacturer of specialist sporting clothes. But, it was not until 1948 that the Le Coq Sportif (LCS) brand was trademarked.

In 1966 LCS entered into a partnership with adidas – LCS introduced adidas to French athletics, while adidas brought its shoe skills and international presence to the table. But after a legal disagreement in 1974, ownership of LCS went to the adidas group. During this time, LCS really developed its training shoe range, and adidas skilfully boosted LCS by adding models associated with new sports.

In 1995 adidas lost control of the group to an American company. This was too much for French pride and three years later a group of contractors from Alsace bought the LCS brand back.

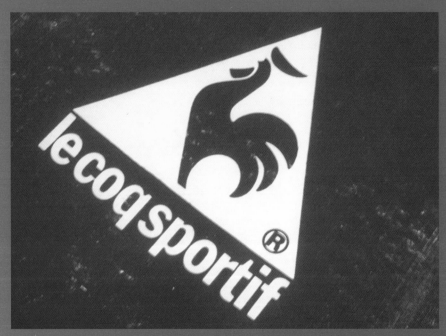

space

It was in 1974 that adidas became owners of this famous French company. German brand expertise allied to French innovation produced some definable Le Coq Sportif models. The Space, seen here, was an early 1980s' issue running shoe with an unmistakable Le Coq feel; note the plastic support with the imprint detail.

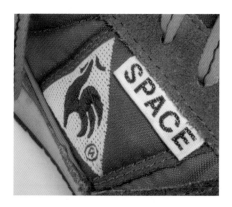

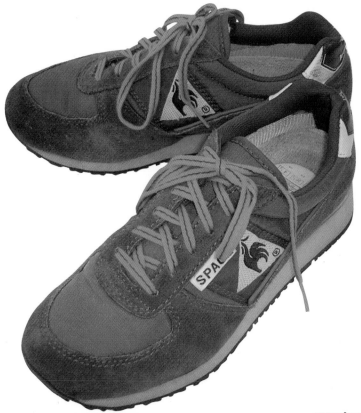

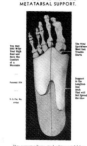
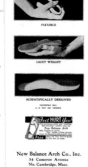
new balance **brand history**

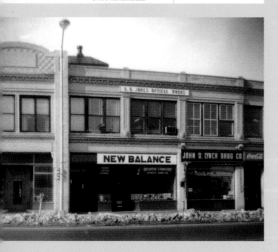

New Balance's reputation comes down to us through its involvement in the New York Marathon – but the story's roots are in Cambridge, Massachusetts, the spiritual home of marathons. Here, in 1906, a 33-year-old English immigrant, William J. Riley, took his first steps into trainer history.

A concern with foot health had led Riley into the field of prescription footwear made with special arch supports. Due to the nature of his shoe production and the 'new balance' it provided for wearers, the company name came into being.

Initial success led Riley, in 1934, into partnership with his leading salesman, Arthur Hall, who had been selling Riley's

ABOVE LEFT This New Balance ad stresses orthopaedic benefits.
LEFT The first New Balance store, in Boston, Massachusetts.

shoes to 'policemen and other folks who were on their feet all day'. It was another six years, however, before New Balance was to make its first forays into the sporting world. Success was gained via Dan McBride, who competed in the Massachusetts Reddish Road Race wearing a pair of black kangaroo-leather running shoes with crepe soles.

In the 1950s the company passed to Riley's relatives, the Kidds, but prescription footwear remained the basis of the company until 1961, when they decided to turn their specialized knowledge to the sports industry. The result was the Trackster, with its unique width fittings and ripple sole. New Balance's reputation had begun to spread to a wider audience.

The modern-day story of New Balance is closely tied to 1972 when, on the day of the Boston Marathon, the company was

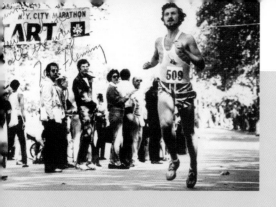

ABOVE Tom Fleming winning the New York Marathon wearing NB 320s.

purchased by Jim Davis. At this point the company was making only 30 models of shoe and had six full-time workers.

In 1975 Tom Fleming won the New York Marathon wearing New Balance model 320 running shoes. Allied to this, New Balance was also voted the number one running shoe in the prestigious *Runner's World* magazine, and it looked as though the company were going to challenge for the number one spot in the training shoe world. However, despite these and other successes, New Balance never quite entered the very highest echelons of training-shoe sales.

Despite this lack of ultimate success, New Balance can be described as a brand that 'punches above its weight'. Although company sales are not as large as some, its reputation means that it always seems to be on the verge of breaking into the top spot. Of all the brands featured in this book, New Balance is, arguably, held in the highest respect by competitors in the field for which the shoes were developed – the running world.

With the aim of making the shoe itself 'the star', the company ethos precludes any high-profile, superstar endorsements. The focus is on research and design, allied to technological innovation and superior manufacturing. In line with this, New Balance training shoes have been made in the Lake District of England since 1982, when other sports shoe companies have shifted production to regions where labour costs are lower. In 2002, the company broke through the one million pair sales barrier for the first time.

As far as 'tribal allegiance' is concerned, New Balance did have a cult following with Football Casuals, when followers in the north-west of England adopted them. Also in the late 1990s the 801 model became popular in fashion circles and the company responded by releasing the model in three new colourways.

A unique feature of New Balance shoes is the use of model numbers rather than names (except for the initial Trackster). The higher the shoe number, the greater its specification. Therefore, the 2000 model is the flagship shoe of the range while the 600 is the entry-level model. The product numbering system can also help to date most shoes. Annual updates are indicated by numerical increments, so that the 852 would become the 853 model the next year it was produced.

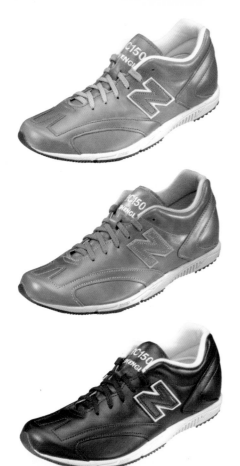

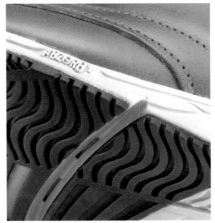

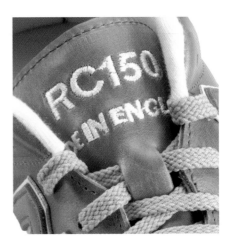

150

This extremely lightweight and responsive racing competition shoe was designed to be suitable for distances up to about 6½ miles (10 km). The version seen here is in its classic leather variety. New Balance has also released it in a new format with 'modern' materials, such as mesh and micro suede.

230

In this example it's possible to see New Balance falling under the influence of the modern 'space-age' design. However, the company has remained true to its sporting roots, and the 230 is a lightweight racing model with 'C-Cap' midsole and spikeless, solid-rubber outsole. It is suitable for cross-country running and indoor and outdoor track events.

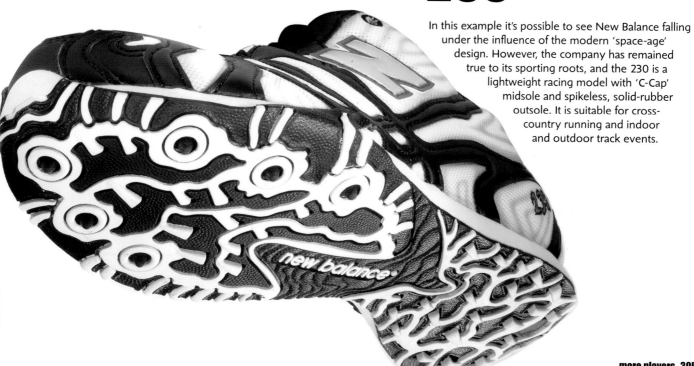

320

The 320 is probably the most lauded of all the New Balance models. It was released in 1975 and, although expensive, was extremely popular and came home the winner in the famous New York Marathon. The highly regarded magazine *Runner's World* named the 320 the best training shoe in 1976.

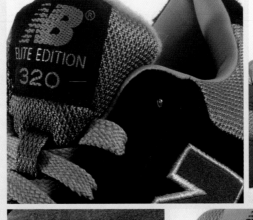

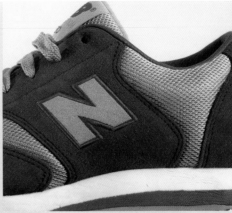

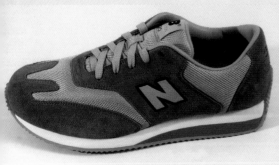

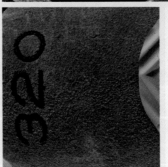

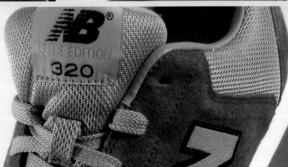

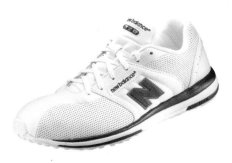

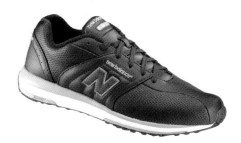

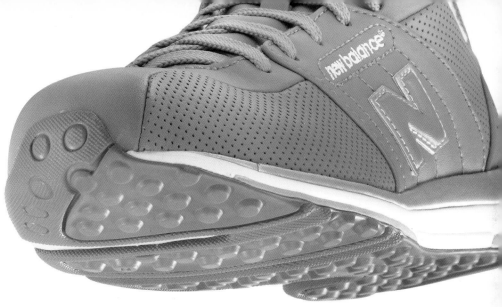

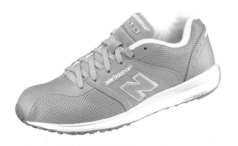

520

The 520 is another of New Balance's long-running models. The example seen here is the modern version made under the banner of the Heritage range. The modern 520 packs in a range of technical features that give it a truly contemporary edge. With New Balance's new 'Abzorb' cushioning, midfoot stability web, and new leather upper it is a classic shoe built for performance.

568

The 568 is one of the older models on offer from New Balance. It was developed as an early short-distance running shoe and has been on sale for some time. Again, it is featured here as part of the latest Heritage range, and uses 'leisure-orientated' colours and materials. The green version is made of suede pigs' leather.

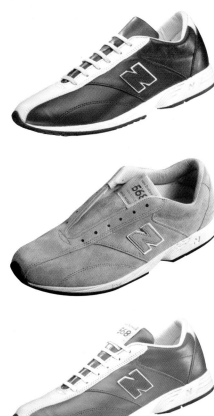

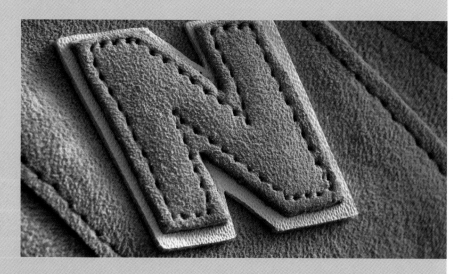

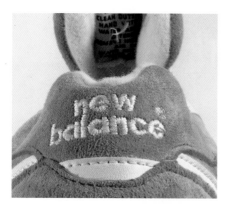

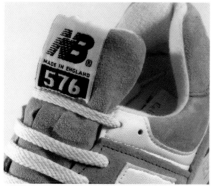

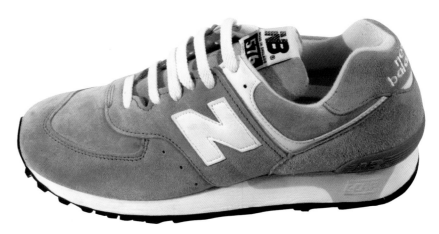

576

As the result of an earlier model, the 675, not selling well, New Balance was left with extra sole units. In 1986, the company decided to change the model name to 576. As well, it altered the colours of the uppers and the materials used and the shoe took off. The spare sole units and many more since were shifted.

577

Knowing as we do that New Balance distinguishes its shoes by numbers rather than names, the 577 is a later model of the 576. The basic model number is the 57 and each year the shoe is reproduced the number goes up in increments (1 usually, as in this case, but sometimes 10). Hence this is a 577, a 576 released a year or two later. However, this version uses basic leather over suede.

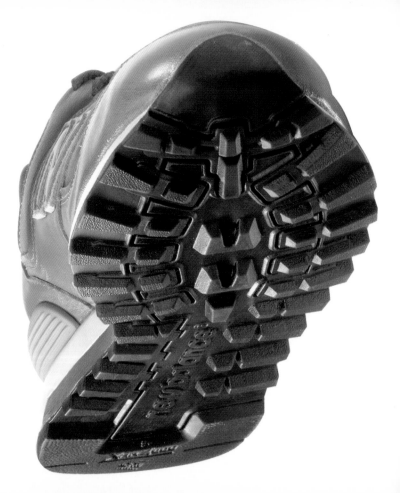

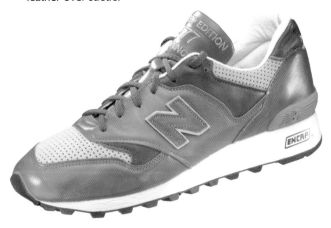

850

The 850 was released as a highly specified walking shoe and it has been given a contemporary feel with modern upper materials and various colourways. These new specifications are an example of how New Balance, along with the other brands, produces designs with the leisure market firmly in mind.

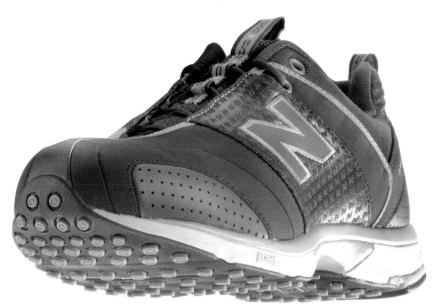

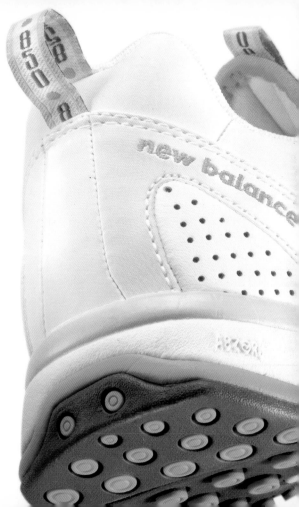

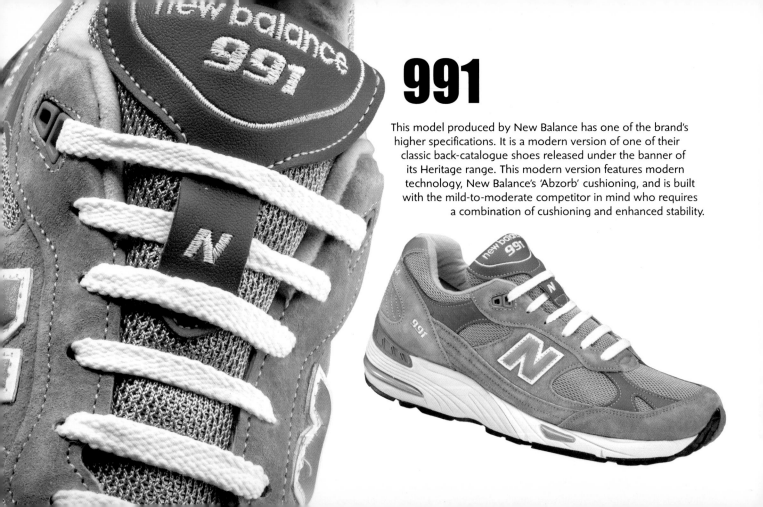

991

This model produced by New Balance has one of the brand's higher specifications. It is a modern version of one of their classic back-catalogue shoes released under the banner of its Heritage range. This modern version features modern technology, New Balance's 'Abzorb' cushioning, and is built with the mild-to-moderate competitor in mind who requires a combination of cushioning and enhanced stability.

996

The 'flagship' shoe for New Balance is the 2000 series. All New Balance models have numbers rather than names, and the basic premise is that the higher the number, the higher the specification of the shoe. Therefore, this 996 is the best specified, in terms of production and materials, that we feature.

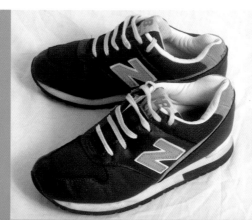
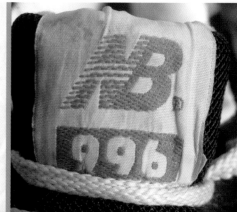
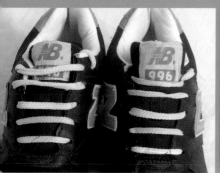
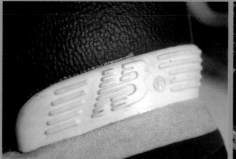
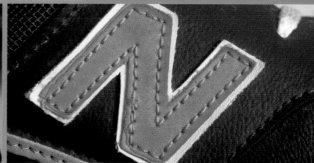

collector

CAMILLA FLOYD, PETER JANSSON & ERIK BÖRJESSON

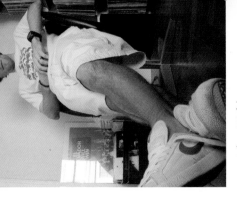

Contrary to popular myth, Scandinavia isn't really clean. Not that it ever stops people playing soccer. Up north it's never too wet, muddy (or late) for a kick-around. You could say we like to get our feet dirty.

Scandinavians have a genuine love for sneakers. When Björn Borg wore his Diadoras, we admired him for his shoes as well as his game. In the 1990s, when the Clydes and Gazelles, and later the Cortez and Air Force 1s, resurfaced, everyone rocked them. People here know sneakers. It's just that they're not too good at taking care of them.

ABOVE Johan Wirfalt, editor of *Bon* magazine, Sweden, interviews three local trainer collectors.

CARMILLA FLOYD

Carmilla is a journalist and writer. Born in Los Angeles but raised in Stockholm, Sweden, she makes regular trips back to East L.A., documenting the Mexican-American community and gang culture.

JW: Why are you into sneakers?

CF: When I was younger, where I lived it was very important to have sneakers that no one else had. Shoes are important, because whatever style you're into, the shoes will give you away.

JW: How many sneakers are in your collection?

CF: I have around six pairs that I wear and 40 that are dead. Usually I get hooked on one pair and wear them every day for months.

JW: Which is your first sneaker memory?

CF: I do remember the first Allen Iversons. I was in New York City and saw a guy on the street in blue leather Iversons. I spent a week trying to find them. In desperation I took a pair of old white Nikes and painted them bright blue. I wore them only once and became a laughing stock.

JW: Which is your best sneaker find?

CF: Many years ago I went on vacation to Puerto Vallarta on the Pacific coast of Mexico. I discovered a sneaker store with a good selection and suddenly I saw a pair of original Air Max 95s on the shelf. There was only one pair left and they were my size!

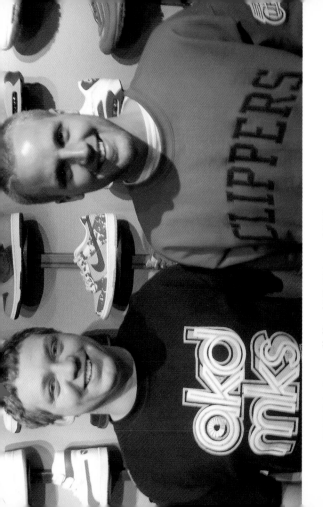

ERIK BÖRJESSON AND PETER JANSSON

Erik and Peter have been buying and selling sneakers for different sport stores in Stockholm since the early 1990s. They opened their own store, Sneakersnstuff, in 1999 and now have two others.

JW: How did you get into sneakers?
EB: I was very into basketball and in 1987 I saw a commercial for Air Jordans in the break in a game recorded from American television.
PJ: I think it was just about wanting to have the freshest kicks in school.

JW: What is it about the hunt for sneakers that is so appealing?
EB: Getting the ones that nobody has seen.
PJ: The chance you may find a pair that you didn't even know existed.

JW: Do you have any rituals around your sneakers?
EB: When I pick up a new pair I lace them and put them by my bed when I go to sleep. If they're really special, they get to stay in the box.
PJ: Not really, just meticulous cleaning with soap, water and Scotchbrite.

JW: You get to name one sneaker model after yourself, which one is it?
EB: A basketball shoe, probably Jordan V.
PJ: Nike Air Flow, definitely.

JW: Can sneakers 'die'?
EB: A shoe is alive as long as you remember you've got it.
PJ: Good sneakers never die. Just look at Chuck Taylors.

P-F flyers

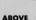

brand history

Rather than being a brand name, the 'P-F' in P-F Flyers stands for 'Posture Foundation'. The story starts in 1900 with B.F. Goodrich, the original parent company and inventor of P-F Flyers. Goodrich was one of 19 companies making canvas and rubber-soled shoes at the time that merged to form U.S. Royal. Developed as a lo-top canvas shoe, the Posture Foundation tag was the selling point drawing attention to Goodrich's claim that P-F Flyers could aid posture when running or walking.

After years of playing second fiddle to brands such as Converse and Pro-Keds, and becoming standard army-issue footwear, P-F Flyers became stuck with a reputation as shoes 'your mum would make you wear'. This, however, changed in 1971 when Converse bought the shoes, and Converse P-F Flyers were born. Converse added some much needed

ABOVE
An original and rare B.F. Goodrich P-F Flyers box.

glamour, but later had to sell off the P-F Flyers brand to settle a U.S. Department of Justice complaint that it had a monopoly share of the sneaker market of the day. Converse had also acquired the B.F. Goodrich Jack Purcell, but this brand it was allowed to keep.

The brand name passed to LJO Inc., who owned the P-F Flyers name from 1991 to 2001. Some P-F Flyers were made, but they looked like a canvas version of the Reebok Freestyle. In February 2001, New Balance acquired the P-F Flyers brand and re-released the shoe in a big way in 2003.

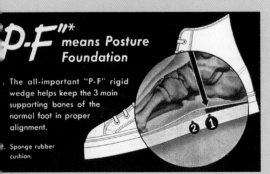

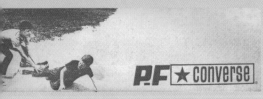

TOP The Posture in P-F explained.
ABOVE A P-F advertisement from the 1970s – an era of Converse ownership.

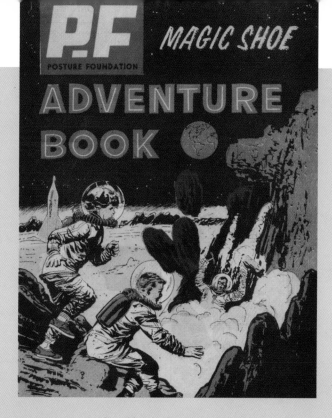

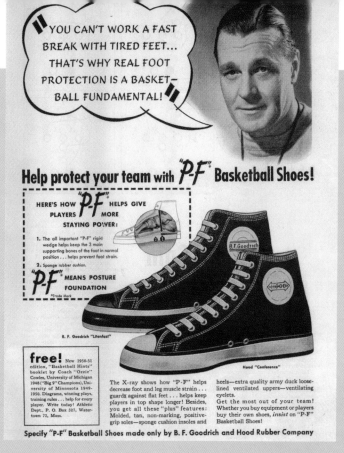

ABOVE Encouraging brand loyalty from an early age.
RIGHT P-F pushing its basketball credentials.

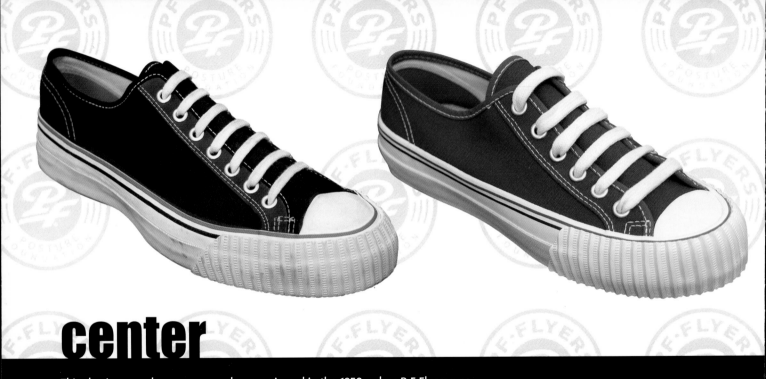

center

This classic general-purpose gym shoe was issued in the 1950s when P-F Flyers was
at the height of its popularity. The Posture Foundation of the shoes was meant to

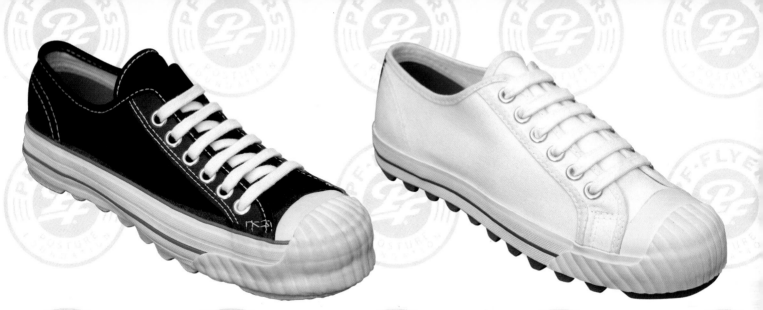

grounder

Here is another 1950s' issue from P-F Flyers, but this shoe was designed more with outdoor sports in mind. To this end, the Grounder had a cleat-like sole that was intended to produce better grip on grass and earth. This is one of the classic shoes on the list to be reissued by New Balance – the brand's current owner.

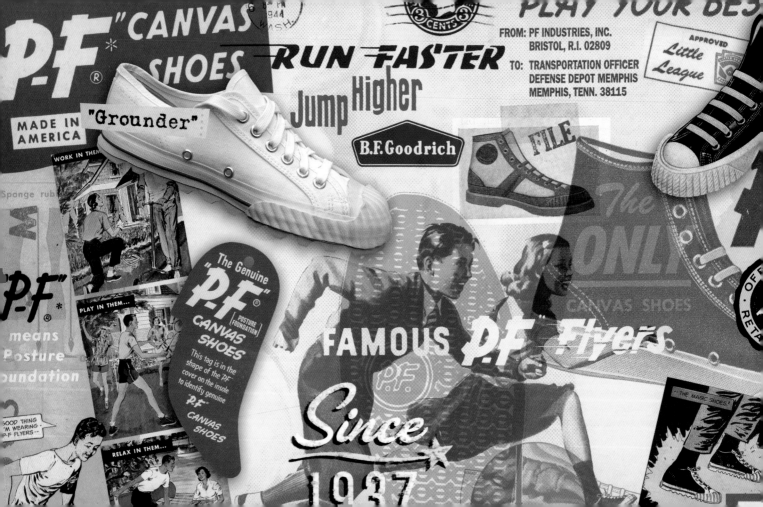

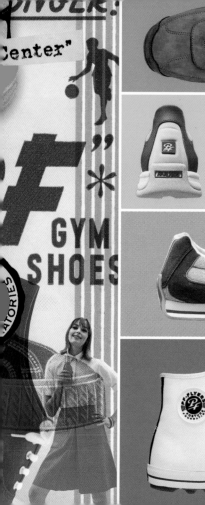

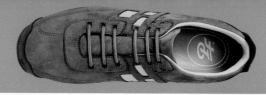

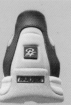

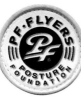

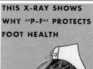

PF·FLYERS POSTURE FOUNDATION

THIS X-RAY SHOWS
WHY "P-F" PROTECTS
FOOT HEALTH

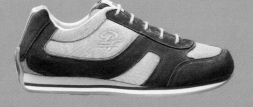

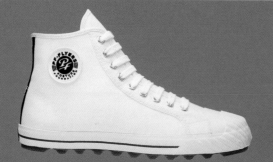

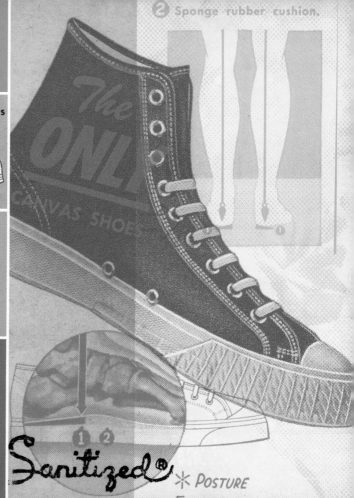

2 Sponge rubber cushion.

The **ONLY**
CANVAS SHOES

Sanitized ✳ POSTURE

pro-keds brand history

The story of this venerable old company began in 1892, the year when the U.S. Rubber Company began producing rubber specifically for use as the soles of shoes. During 1916, U.S. Rubber merged with tyre giant Charles Goodyear and started making rubber-soled, hi-top shoes known as Keds (*see pages 40–1*).

However, it was not until 1949 that the now far better-known name of Pro-Keds appeared on the scene. It was in this year that Keds developed its original athletic line of shoes, which was aimed primarily at basketball players. However, this new range looked so similar to the Converse All Star that, to be honest, the design must be thought of as one of the first examples of sports emulation. In order to make the difference between the two products a little more obvious, Keds developed its distinctive, triple-striped side sole.

With its specialist shoes now established with the Pro-Keds name, the company was quick to latch on to the potential of sporting endorsement. Thus, Pro-Keds was endorsed by five-times world champion Minneapolis Lakers centre, George Mikan, the first truly 'big man' in the National Basketball Association (NBA).

During the 1960s the trainer brands really started to grow, but by the 1970s, even with the booming popularity of running, Pro-Keds had slipped behind. It was bought by the Stride Rite corporation and the shoes were from then built more with comfort than speed in mind.

Recently, New Balance acquired the rights to Pro-Keds originals and they are due to be reissued in the near future.

RIGHT This advertisement for hi- and lo-top Pro-Keds dates from 1978.

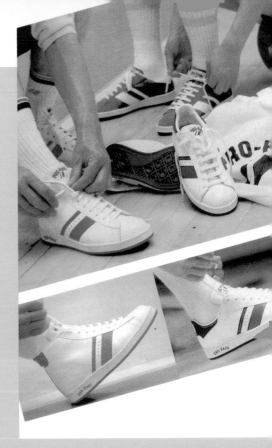

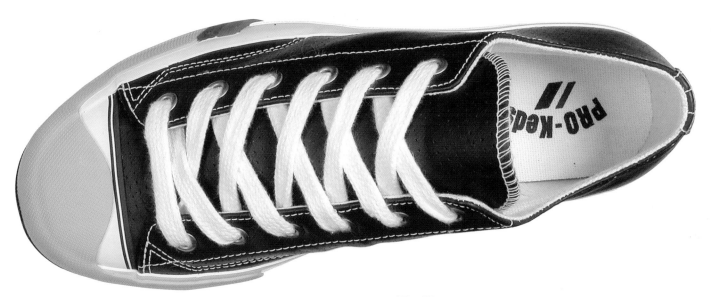

court king

The Court King is one of the oldest and most famous of all Pro-Keds. Designed as a basketball shoe, a fact reflected in the name, the model has many of the Pro-Keds signatures – two stripes on the side sole and the very recognizable rubber-toe design. The upper is full-grain leather and sole unit is natural rubber.

court king triple strap

The Court King Triple Strap is the same basic shoe as the Court King in design and specification; however, Pro-Keds (along with other makers) incorporated straps to achieve a better fit and to provide support for the foot. Unlike the laced Court King, which comes in numerous colourways, the Triple Strap comes in only three.

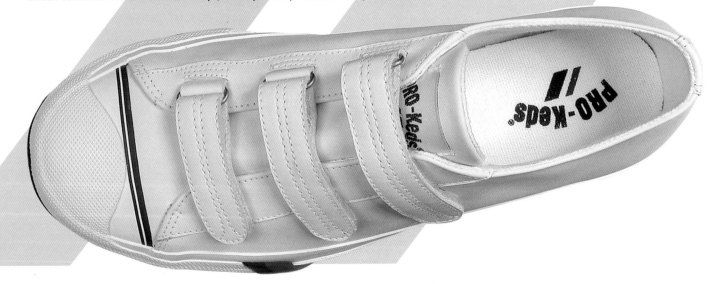

royal master

The Royal Master is a later issue from Pro-Keds and aimed to provide a better overall specification and extra foot protection for basketball players. The shoe, which has been reissued recently, comes in either full-grain leather or suede versions. Pro-Keds had listened to basketball players and so developed a chunky padded sole to alleviate friction.

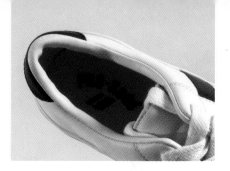

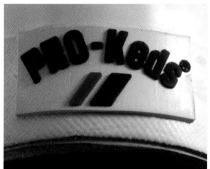

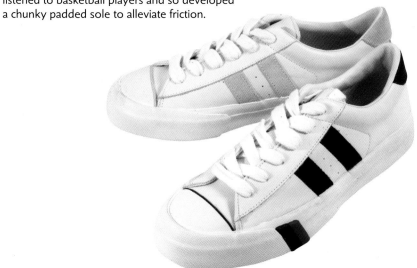

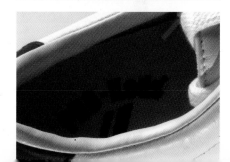

saucony brand history

Saucony's roots go back to Abraham Hyde, a cobbler and Russian immigrant to Massachusetts, U.S.A., who opened a shoe shop in 1910. The company prospered as A. R. Hyde and Sons and eventually developed the production of a range of athletic shoes. During the 1960s the company worked with NASA and the boots worn by the first astronaut to walk in space carried the Hyde label.

In 1968, Hyde decided to expanded by acquiring the Saucony Shoe Manufacturing Company of Pennsylvania. But Saucony's running shoes remained the closely kept secret of a small group of serious runners until 1977, when one of its shoes was recognized with a best-quality award by a top U.S. magazine. The resulting publicity established Saucony's name and its reputation for high quality and innovative technical performance for which it is known today.

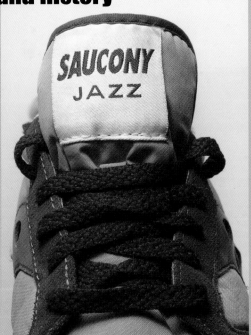
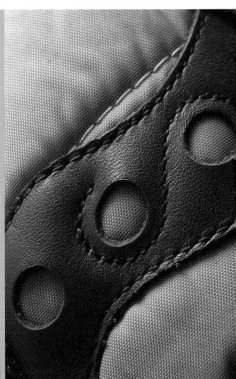

jazz

The Jazz is the best known of all Saucony shoes. The development of the company's sneakers was heavily influenced by the popularity of long-distance and marathon running, and runners clad in Saucony Jazz performed well, gaining the acclaim of *Runner's World* magazine and establishing this model as a serious running shoe.

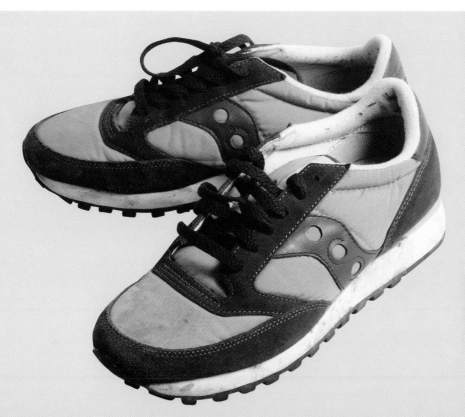

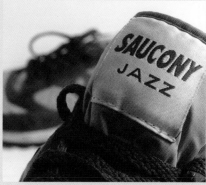

vans brand history

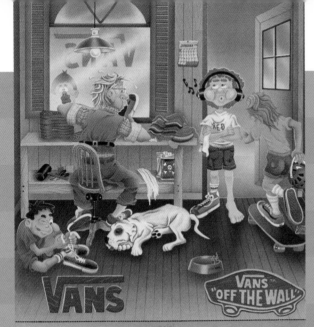

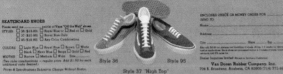

The original 'off the Wall' Vans certainly looked distinctive and the history of the company is far from being a usual one. A revealing story from the early days helps to illustrate this point. When Paul Van Doren opened his shop in California in 1966, shoes were priced at $2.49 and $4.99. There was a slight problem – he didn't keep any pennies to give people as change when they bought his shoes. So, instead of simply keeping the small amount of change, he gave them their shoes and asked each to come back and pay the next day.

And guess what? They all came back and paid (apparently).

Anyway, true or not, the founder of the company, Paul Van Doren (hence, the Vans name) and his three partners had established their company to manufacture canvas shoes for direct sale to the public through locally based, company-owned outlets. In this way, they hoped to cut margins by removing the middleman's takings. The company was using the now ancient vulcanization method of production, in which the rubber is bonded to canvas in huge oven chambers. This resulted in the distinctive style that became the signature look of the company. The vulcanization process produced extremely thick soles, which made them difficult to destroy and so endeared them to the skateboarding fraternity, who were always looking for shoes to stand up to hard knocks.

As well as the penny change story, the company took its approach to customer care to extremes. Up until the early 1980s (before Paul Van Doren and partners sold the company in 1988), Vans used to make custom shoes – and when Van Doren said custom, he meant custom.

Long before Nike's modern approach to on-line customization, anybody buying a pair of Vans could specify literally how the shoes were to come. You could have the left one green and purple, say, and the right one orange and blue. You could even supply your own fabric, and the company would cover your shoes in it. And it didn't stop there – Vans also offered a range of printed images to put on the sides of the soles, and as a result many early Vans have rainbows, hearts or checks on them.

However, it was during the early 1970s, with the skateboarding craze sweeping California, that Vans became a 'must

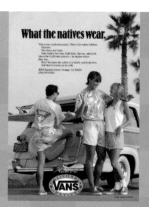 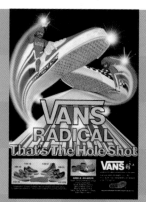 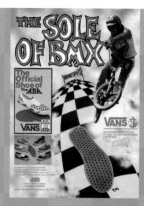

ABOVE These ads (from left to right) are aimed at the surf, skate and BMX crazes.

have' for anybody with a board. Later, BMX riders started wearing Vans, which gave the shoes the advertising slogan 'The Sole of BMX'. The company continued to grow steadily through the 1970s, but it wasn't until 1980, when Jeff Spicoli (played by Sean Penn), the ultimate California surfer, wore a pair of black-and-white checked Vans in the now classic movie *Fast Times at Ridgemont High*, that the Vans craze went nationwide. At this point, Vans took off and demand rapidly outstripped supply.

The company went off the rails when Paul Van Doren left in 1980, but he was brought back on board three years later, since when Vans has reinvented itself as the successful brand we know today.

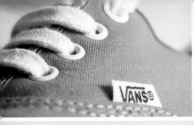
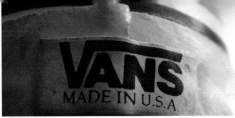
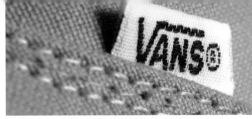

authentic

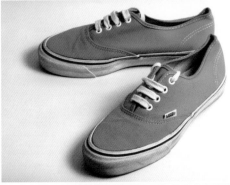

Paul Van Doren and his three partners opened their first shoe store at 704 East Broadway, Anaheim, California, on 16 March 1966. The Van Doren Rubber Company was unusual in that it not only manufactured shoes, it also sold them directly to the public. On their first morning, 12 customers purchased shoes, which were made that day and were ready to be picked up in the afternoon. Those shoes were the Vans deck shoes 44, now known as the Authentic.

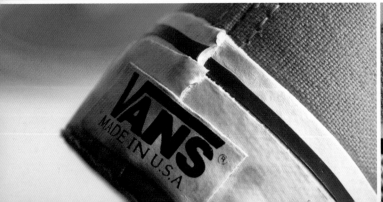
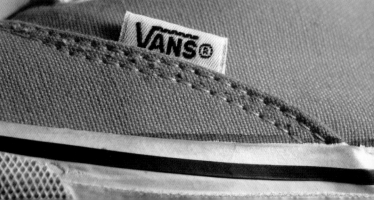

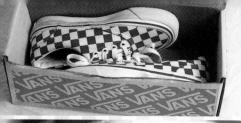
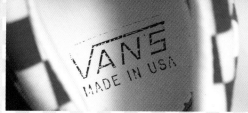
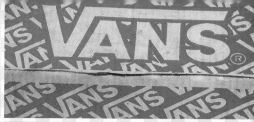
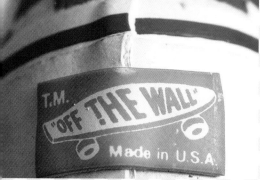

VANS
ORANGE, CA. 92665 ®

95-XX-4004
WS17593

2

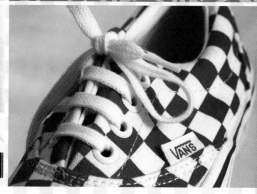
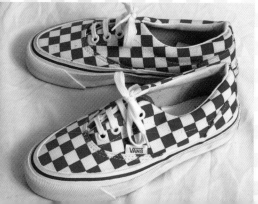

era checkerboard

Skateboarders in the early 1970s appreciated Vans' cheap price, rugged construction, and sticky sole. In 1976 the company brought in Tony Alva and Stacy Peralta to design shoes specifically with skate in mind. This resulted in a padded collar and different colourways and Vans 95, now known as the Era Checkerboard, was born.

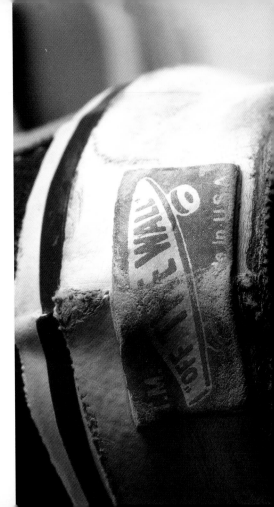

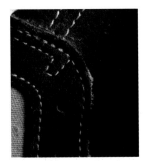

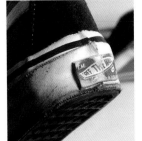

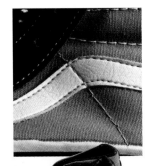

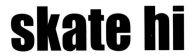

skate hi

As time went on, skateboarders were having much more of an input into the design of the Vans range. Flying out of concrete pools at high speed was taking its toll on skaters' feet, so when they wanted a hi-top with more ankle protection, Vans developed the first enclosed, padded, hi-top skate shoe called the Skate Hi, sometimes written as the SK8 Hi, to satisfy this need.

slip-on

This model is, arguably, the most frequently seen and well known of the Vans range. The Slip-On model was part of the Era design and it was first introduced in 1979. With the help of skateboarders and BMX riders, it soon become the rage in southern California. In 1982 the Vans Slip-On gained international attention and appeal when the shoe was worn by Sean Penn in the movie *Fast Times at Ridgemont High*. Today, these shoes are seen all over the world in myriad colours and styles.

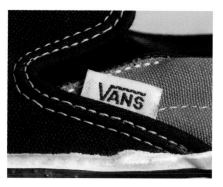

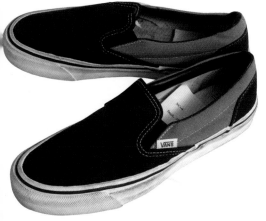

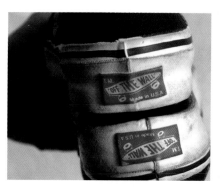

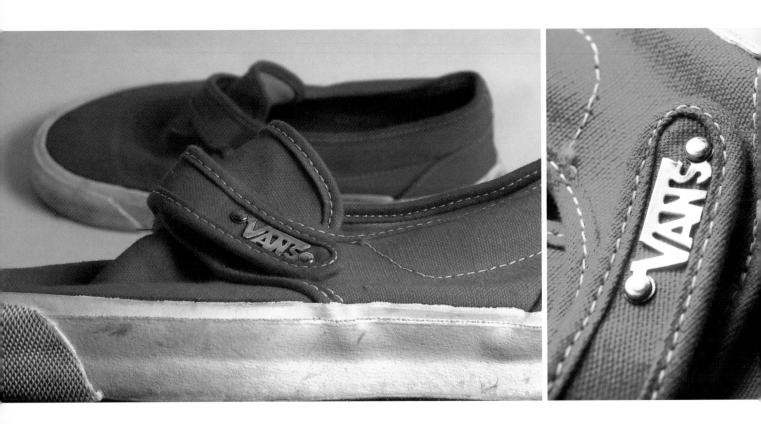

strap

Here we see another variation on the classic Vans deck shoe, and this model is particularly rare. Vans did its own take on the Velcro strap, to provide ease of use and a more comfortable fit. Vans paid attention to detail, and the Flying Vans logo can be seen in polished metal on the early models of this design.

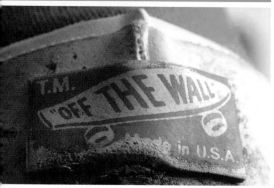

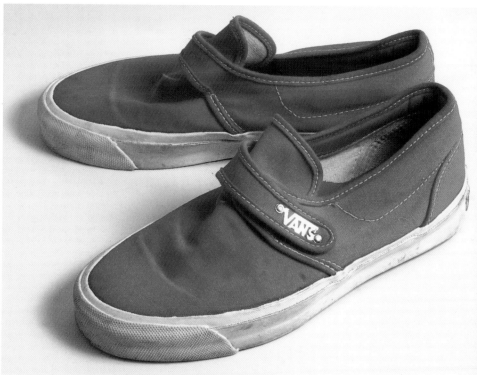

collector
BRYAN WHALEN

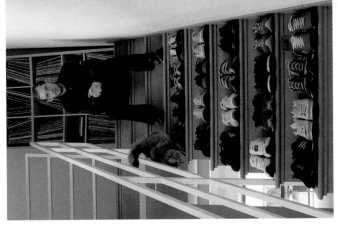

Bryan Whalen is the label manager at Look Records in San Francisco, California, and an avid trainer fan and collector.

'I get this call from a friend saying, "Hey, will you write some stuff about sneakers?" To which I reply, "Well . . . I guess, but what do you want me to say?". What could possibly be said that hasn't been said a million times before? Except, maybe . . . perhaps . . .

I might've mentioned my first memories of wanting anything other than a G.I. Joe action figure, my first pair of Jordans. Or, maybe I'd recall the summer I got my fluorescent yellow and baby blue Aqua Socks. They were perfect in that 100-degree-plus weather. It was like being barefoot without the asphalt burns. Perfect for stomping through local creeks/ drainage ditches/sewer tunnels. By the time summer camp rolled around, they were more or less broken in, with the only hole limited to the left pinky toe. That didn't last long. Two weeks of mud, rocks, campfires, canoes, dead snakes, chlorine, bug repellant and miles of running had taken their toll. The shoes were less shoe, more hole. Aromatically, well, when my parents picked me up, I had to ride with my feet out of the window. We didn't even go home. It was straight to the local Foot Locker. My parents asked me what I wanted to replace my pieces of neoprene and rubber. "Aqua Socks, of course!"

Those are the type of things I could have written. My Budweiser/Spuds McKenzie Hawaiian Print Vans. The summer I ran away and a skinhead gave me some Jordan VIs he'd "acquired". The Wallabees I stole from my friend's senile grandfather. I could even write about my collection of re-issues just to annoy the trainer purists. These are the types of thing I could expound on. Unfortunately, they aren't very relevant to anyone else, except me. What's the big deal anyway? It's just shoes, right? I was simply left thinking, "What the hell can I write about?"'

collector
CHRIS HALL

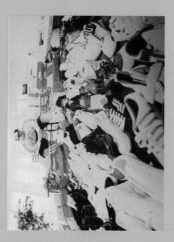

Sneaker collector Chris Hall is an ex-professional skater and now works as a footwear culture consultant.

NH: How do you see skaters' love for their shoes?

CH: I guess back in the early 1980s skaters were mostly in Vans. I do remember Tony Alva and his crew in Nike Bruins with the fat 'Swooshes'. They must have been mad cheap back then and grippy on the board. I remember you used to be able to order custom vans in any style, colour, and design you wanted. I never ordered any and regret it to this day. In 1984–86 I remember basketball shoes being skated in a lot. Gonz in AJ 1's – he would paint his all custom and stuff. Then I started wearing AJ 1s and haven't stopped to this day.

NH: Who were your heroes when you started skating?

CH: I began skating in 1983–84. Mark Gonzales influenced me greatly – Gonz is the best skater ever. End of story.

NH: Can you remember your first pair of trainers?

CH: I guess the first pair I really cared about were Air Jordan 85s. Red, black and white. And baby blue and white ones for my boy. Picked up 4 pairs each for $15 a pair in a close-out sale.

NH: Was it love at first site or did they grow on you?

CH: It was kind of mixed. I loved the AJ 1s when they came out. I would actually take some pairs and cut the hi-top part off to make lo tops because they sometimes felt too high on my shins when skating.

NH: Were you an instant addict?

CH: No. I didn't get really hooked until about 1996. And yes I collect. I have about 200 pairs deadstock.

NH: All brands or any one in particular?

CH: I collect a lot of brands, not just Nike or adidas. Stuff like Troop, Converse, Asics, Reebok and New Balance. If it is vintage deadstock, I'll collect it.

vision brand history

The Vision story is down to one man, Brad Dorfman. During the early 1970s in southern California, Dorfman saw the need for more products based around the new style of skating, and in 1976 Vision Skateboards was born. Dorfman brought many skaters on board, including Mark 'the Gonz' Gonzales, who pushed the Vision Skateboard Team to new heights.

It was in 1988 that Vision Street Wear Shoes was born. At the time, except for Vans, skateboarders had no shoe brands of their own. Then came Vision Shoes, footwear designed by skaters who owned and formed the company, using colours and prints to give skateboarders a style of their own. Love them or hate them, you can't ignore them.

RIGHT By Skaters for Skaters, Vision's 1980s' Street Wear logo.

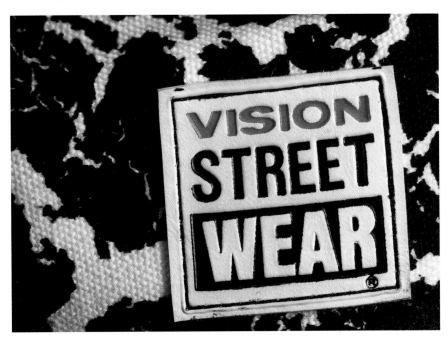

crackle

The Crackle is one of the hi-top skate shoes that were developed by Vision with skating specifically in mind. The shoes featured extra stitching, extra ankle support, and they were particularly known for having the first 'ollie pad' – a small piece of rubber on the shoe designed to help extend shoe life. The Crackle was one of the range to feature Op Art designs and wild colours.

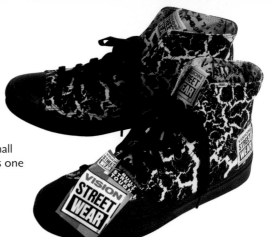

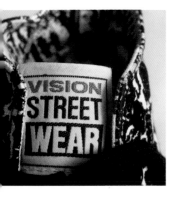

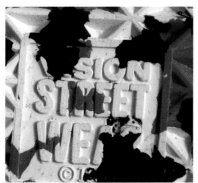

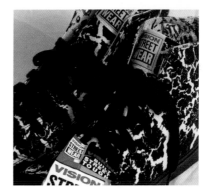

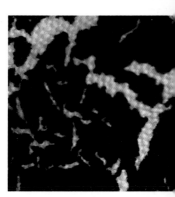

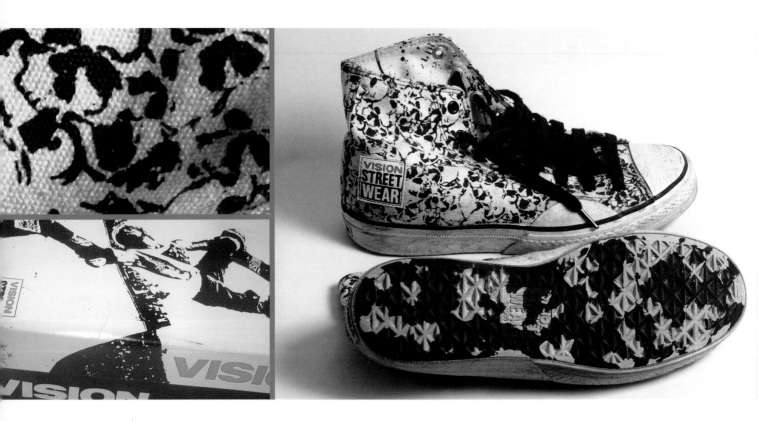

punk skull

This hi-top skate shoe was issued from from 1988 and features all the skate attributes, including infamous 'ollie pad'. The Punk Skull is probably the most collectable and quietest of Vision's skate-shoe designs and was meant to convey a sense of freedom and give the entire line of shoes an image distinct from the 'hippie', 'surf' and 'disco' fashions.

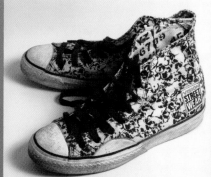

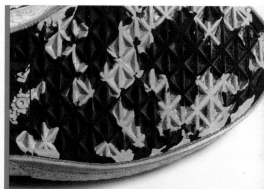

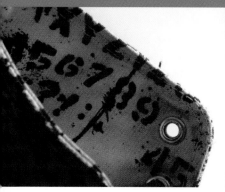

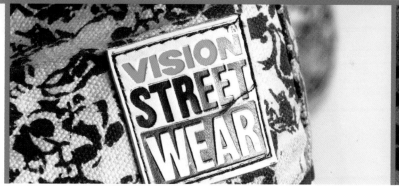

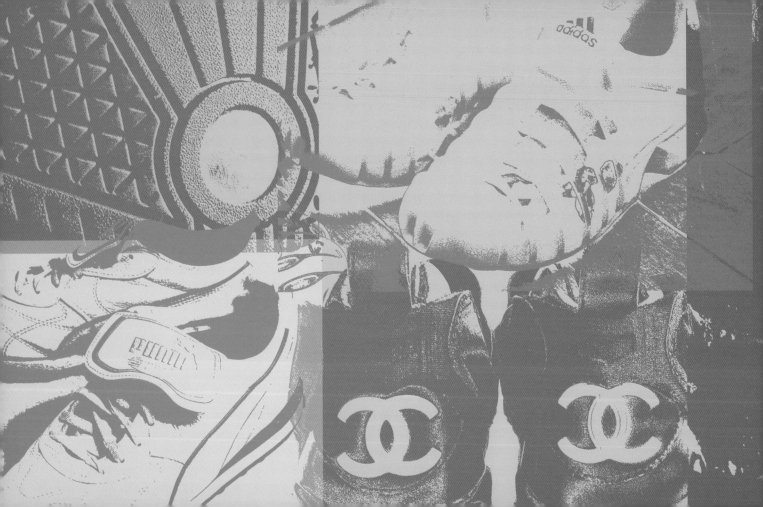

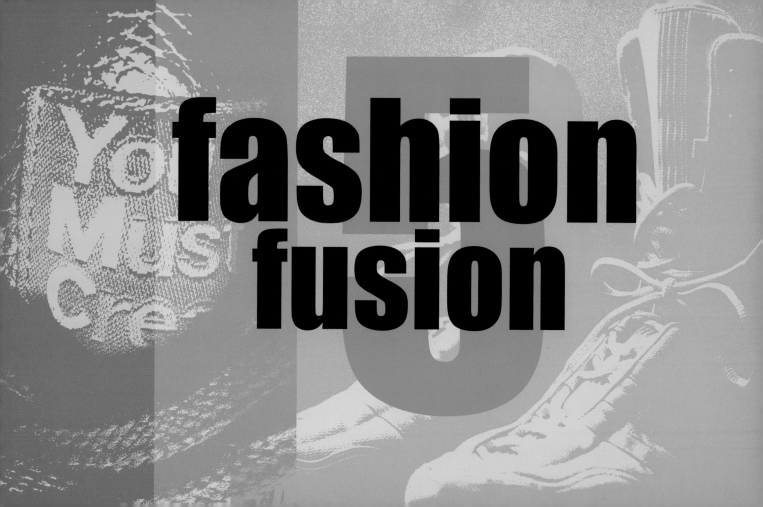

fashion
fusion

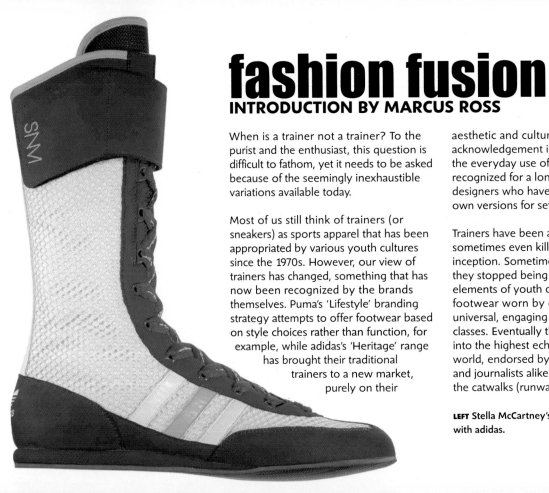

fashion fusion
INTRODUCTION BY MARCUS ROSS

When is a trainer not a trainer? To the purist and the enthusiast, this question is difficult to fathom, yet it needs to be asked because of the seemingly inexhaustible variations available today.

Most of us still think of trainers (or sneakers) as sports apparel that has been appropriated by various youth cultures since the 1970s. However, our view of trainers has changed, something that has now been recognized by the brands themselves. Puma's 'Lifestyle' branding strategy attempts to offer footwear based on style choices rather than function, for example, while adidas's 'Heritage' range has brought their traditional trainers to a new market, purely on their

aesthetic and cultural merit. This acknowledgement is a recent thing, but the everyday use of trainers has been recognized for a long time by fashion designers who have been creating their own versions for several years.

Trainers have been adored, worshipped, sometimes even killed for, since their inception. Sometime in the mid 1990s, they stopped being worn just by certain elements of youth culture and became footwear worn by everybody, truly universal, engaging all ages, trends and classes. Eventually they found their way into the highest echelons of the fashion world, endorsed by designers, models, and journalists alike. For a frenzied while, the catwalks (runways) of Milan and Paris

LEFT Stella McCartney's collaboration with adidas.

awash with the latest 'Swoosh' and 'Brand With Three Stripes'. Fashion by its very nature is cyclical; trends come and go, but the almost obligatory uniform of combat pants and trainers that was the style of the greater part of the 1990s seems to have left an indelible impression on designer fashion.

This more louche approach to dressing up has led many designers to de-formalize parts of their collections, hoping to attract some of this new market. Although fashion designers have flirted with the 'everymans' footwear in the past (Chanel, Dirk Bikkembergs and Walter Van Beirendonck to name just three), the revolution in designer trainers was really kick started in the late 1990s. And this revolution appears

RIGHT The 'own-label' trainer offering from fashion house Chanel.

to have happened in different ways. Large designer names have created their own versions aimed to compete directly in the market created by the sportswear brands, such as Nike and adidas. Dolce & Gabbana who, in comparison to their Italian counterparts, are synonymous with youth and leisure, have combined contemporary sportswear colourways with retro (particularly Italian) styles to create their own take on the trainer.

Alongside the younger Italian brand stands Donna Karan's younger diffusion line, DKNY, which is a symbol of the vibrant energy of its city's namesake. It is unsurprising that an

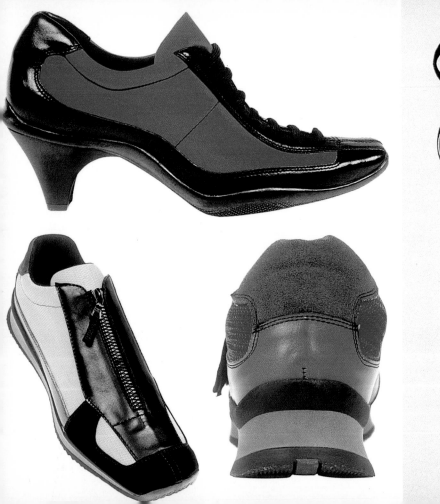
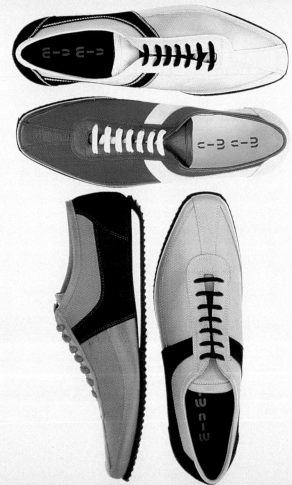

American label should be so successful in this arena, considering American fashion's longstanding relationship with sportswear. Not only have modern sports and music stars made sports apparel fashionable, older American fashion designers, particularly Claire McCardell, pioneered the crossover of sports and leisure wear. Today the DKNY label is stocked in specialist trainer shops alongside the original sports labels.

Collaborations have become commonplace in the world of fashion. The first really recognizable collaboration between sportswear and high fashion was between the German designer Jil Sander and German sports brand Puma. The story goes that Jil Sander wanted the models to wear a football boot, the Puma King, for one of her fashion shows. Puma offered to put a trainer shoe sole on the upper, so they would be practical on the catwalk (runway). Jil Sander then asked if she could put her name to it and retail it. Hence this collaboration between fashion and sport was born, one that still exists, despite the fact that she no longer works at the company that bears her name. Today, Puma also collaborates with Italian-based British designer Neil Barrett, who has discarded laces and enlarged soles in some of his designs. Previously, American giant Converse collaborated with British designer John Richmond, and today Converse works with young American designer John Varvatos. Reebok has worked with Paul Smith on a range of trainers for a few years now, as well as him producing sports-influenced shoes under his own brand name. Perhaps the most interesting of these collaborations is between adidas and Yohji Yamamoto, the iconic Japanese fashion designer. For his Spring–Summer 2001 collection Yamamoto created a collection of sophisticated

OPPOSITE Various trainer-inspired footwear from Italian fashion house Prada.
RIGHT Football boots from Belgian designer Dirk Bikkembergs.

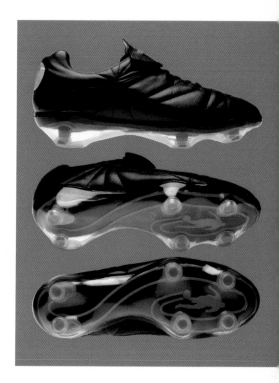

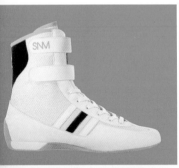

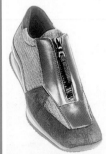

FAR LEFT Stella McCartney's work with adidas.
LEFT Prada's 'trainer-inspired' shoe.
BELOW LEFT Converse All Stars designed by John Varvatos.
RIGHT TOP AND BOTTOM Paul Smith's work with fellow British brand Reebok.
BELOW Neil Barrett's offering in collaboration with Puma.

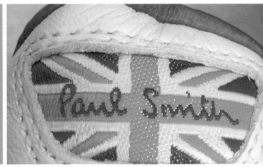

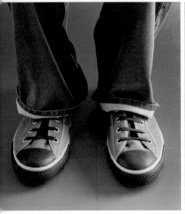

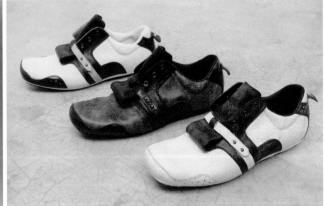

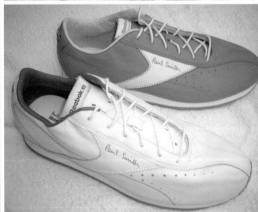

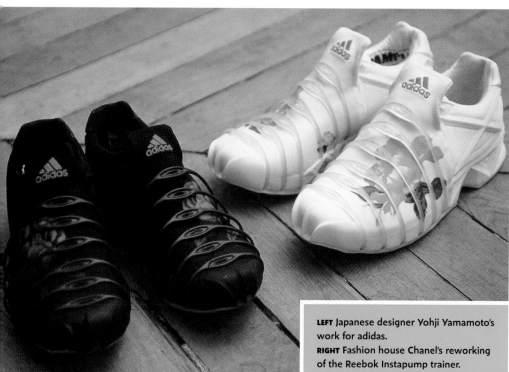

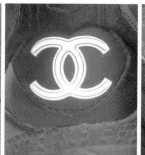

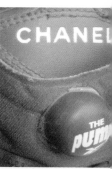

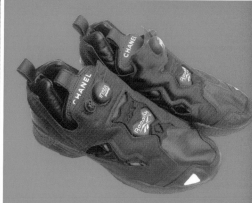

LEFT Japanese designer Yohji Yamamoto's work for adidas.
RIGHT Fashion house Chanel's reworking of the Reebok Instapump trainer.

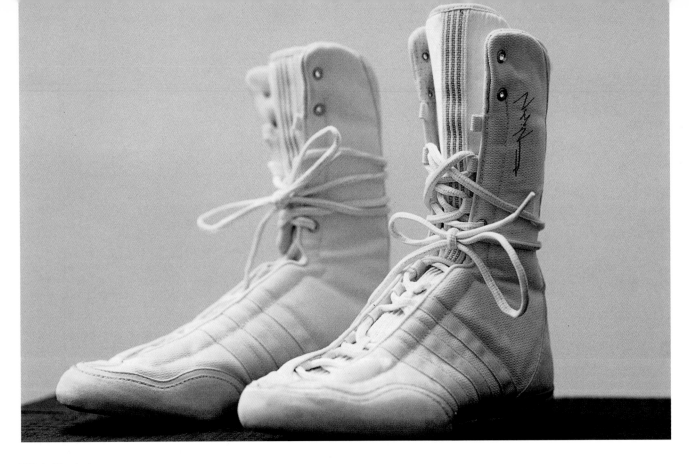

sportswear. That is to say, clothes that were heavily influenced by sportswear in terms of fabric and styling, yet without any sports functionality. Allegedly influenced by the all-encompassing image of adidas's three-stripe logo adorning Tokyo kids, he chose to integrate their logo into the clothes. This led to range of trainers designed by Yohji Yamamoto for adidas. This differed from other collaborations because the shoes were designed from scratch rather than changing existing designs, giving Yamamoto total creative freedom. This was no doubt the first time large, bold flower prints appeared on trainers. In 2002 the two companies created a new clothing label, Y-3, bringing together the disparate influences of sportswear and design.

Elsewhere, fashion designers have tapped into the wealth of history that now exists in trainer design, and used it to create their own breed of footwear. Sometimes this is the downright simple, possibly a mere homage, such as Helmut Lang's leather Converse look-a-likes. (Currently it is very hard to find a genuine pair of leather Jack Purcells.) In the case of Prada, this has been an opportunity to create some of the boldest footwear of the last decade. Standing quite comfortably between radical design and pure commerciality, Prada has produced every type of shoe, including heels that have appropriated both sportswear design and fabric. The influences of sportswear and fashion design are probably best personified by the silver Prada Sport trainer of a few years ago that, curiously, was designed out of function, yet became a style choice that possibly even eschewed Nike and adidas for a brief moment.

OPPOSITE Yohji Yamamoto's Court boxing shoes.
RIGHT More 'conventional' offerings from the Japanese designer with adidas.

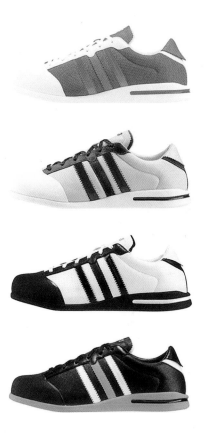

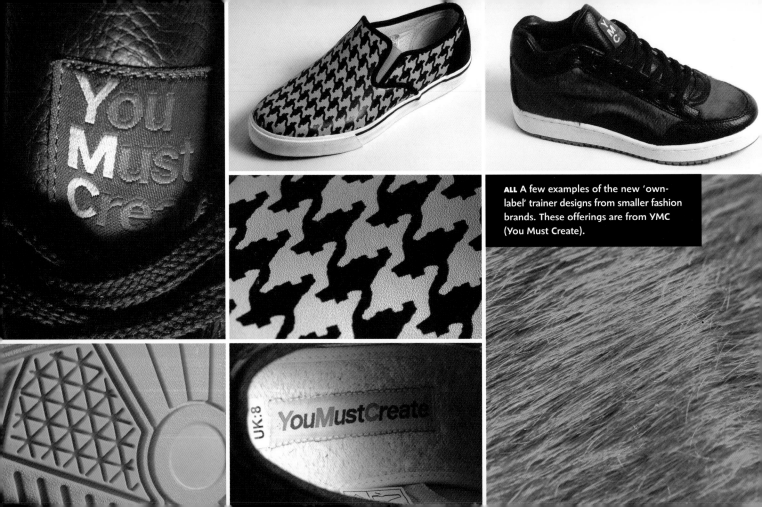

ALL A few examples of the new 'own-label' trainer designs from smaller fashion brands. These offerings are from YMC (You Must Create).

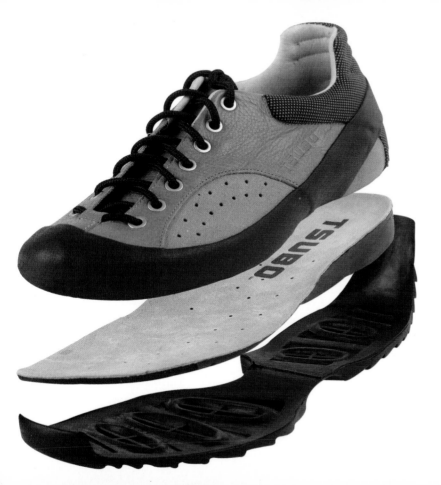

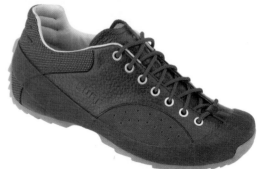

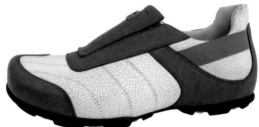

LEFT AND TOP Tsubo is one of several shoe manufacturers to cater for the retro-style sneaker market. Here is the Xeric in leather and suede.
ABOVE Tsubo's Auriga model.

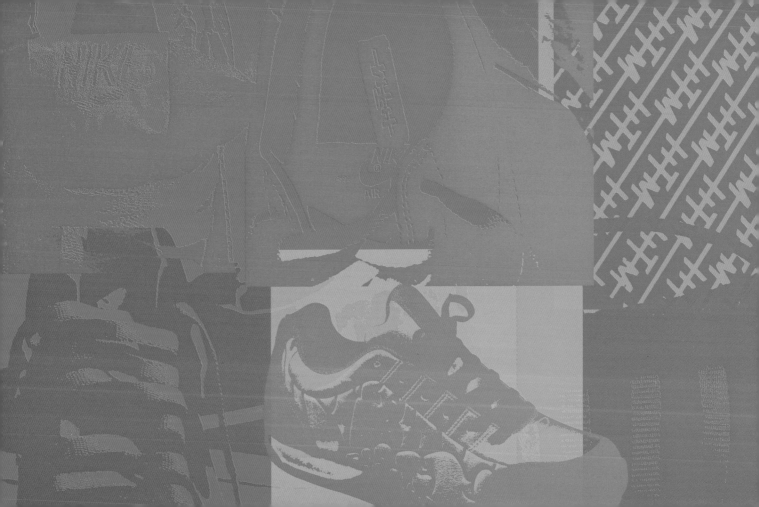

6 collaborations

collaborations
INTRODUCTION

A change is as good as a rest

Although I've never really been into the concept of trainer collaborations, I have had to rethink my position – at least just a little. As you must have noted by this stage in the book, the humble trainer has progressed a long way. It has gone from being a purely functional sporting product, known to relatively few people, to being part of popular culture as a whole. It has found its way into virtually every home and street in the world. No longer is it seen as one thing or another. In this new world, the trainer is as much a fashion accessory as an athletic shoe.

With almost perpetual growth over the past twenty or so years, it would seem that the appetite of the trainer-buying

RIGHT HTM with Nike's Air Force 1 Lo.

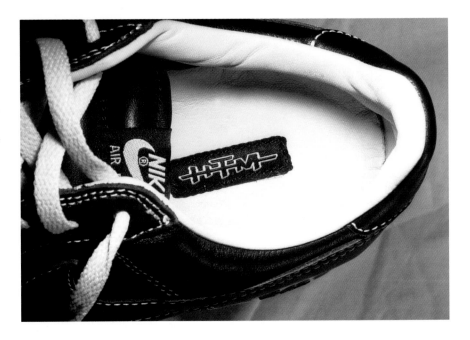

public would have to stall. With this in mind, the brands have busied themselves searching out every avenue to keep their market share on an upward trend.

As sport, leisure, and fashion have fused, so trainer brands have been quick to seek new avenues to exploit. And just as the trainer brands have looked for new openings, so elements of the fashion industry have admired many of the training shoe brands.

In business circles, this is called 'fit' – two separate entities coming together to create improvements for all concerned. It is not surprising, then, that we are seeing more of this 'cross pollination' between trainer brands and other organizations. This is not entirely a new concept – take, for example, the early collaboration between Vans and United Artists in developing a Snoopy-covered Vans hi-top skate shoe (*see page 365*) – and the phenomenon is becoming more common all the time.

While hunting for new opportunities, the brands – with Nike in the lead – have forged modern collaborations. These include Nike's association with the streetwear label Stussy, with whom they collaborated to create the Stussy Dunks. But Nike is also keen to enter what is for them a new market – skatewear. Not alone, Nike has looked on as skate has grown into a massive industry, and recently the company has worked with smaller skate brands, such as Chocolate, in developing a 'skate-orientated' range of Nike shoes.

With hindsight, we all could have predicted the jogging boom in the 1970s and the fitness craze of the 1980s. But only a few did at the time. Times change, and the trainer

RIGHT Vans' collaboration with the fashion company Silas.

brands have changed along with them. It seems that we are in the throes of the birth of a new era for trainers. Perhaps these collaborations, which may seem trivial to 'traditional' sneaker fans, are the new future. Or is it just a fad that will pass? We will have to wait and see, but in the meantime here are some examples of the new collaborations so that you can judge for yourself.

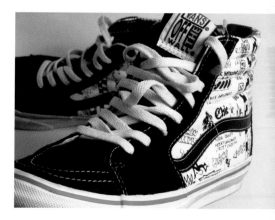

stussy blazer mid

In order to produce this model, Nike has teamed up with the street fashion label Stussy, a company that was traditionally linked to the surf and skate scenes but has now become an integral part of the urban wardrobe. In this 2002 example, Stussy reworked Nike's 'old skool' classic, the Blazer, giving it a modern image by incorporating neon-coloured Swoosh logos.

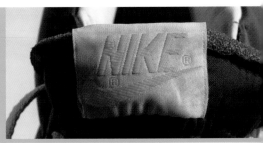

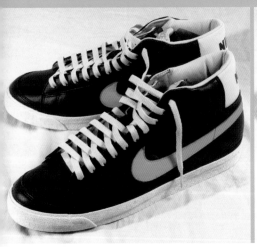

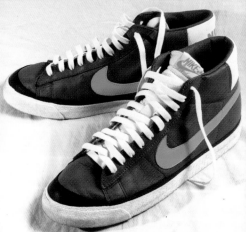

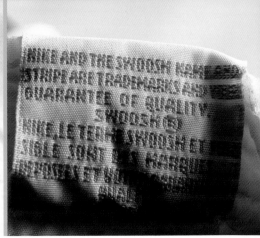

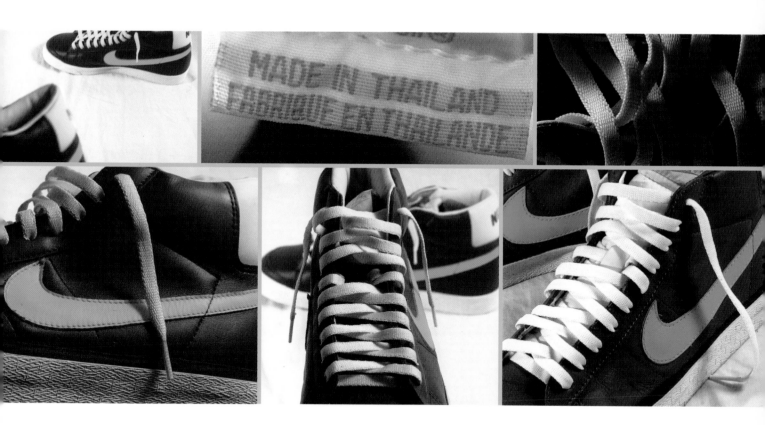

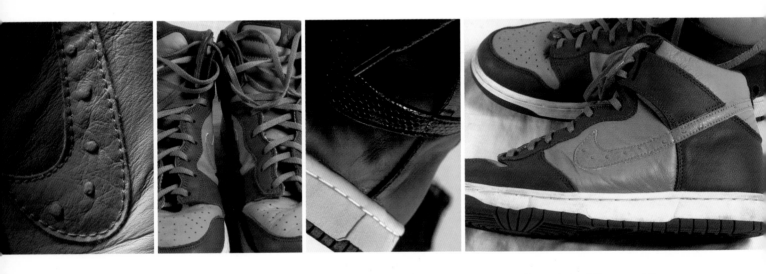

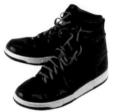 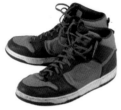

stussy dunk hi plus

This 2002 Dunk Hi Plus collaboration sees Stussy taking an almost opposite approach compared with the Blazer (*see pages 358–9*). With the Blazer, they made a quiet design loud; here, Stussy took the traditionally bright Dunk and toned the shoe right down using muted colourways and fake crocodile and snakeskin material for the Swoosh.

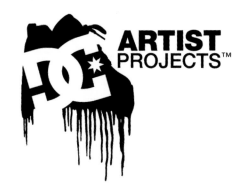

ARTIST PROJECTS™
dc shoes

DC Shoes is a skate shoe company that has invited select artists to collaborate with them on its Artist Projects line of footwear. Each artist is given creative control over the design, branding and packaging of a shoe. The Swift Obey is a collaboration between DC and Shepard Fairey; the Kinsey Coda is named after the artist's version of the Coda shoe; while the 'premier' artist Kaws has reworked the Gauge shoe.

LEFT TO RIGHT The Swift Obey, the Kinsey Coda and the Kaws.

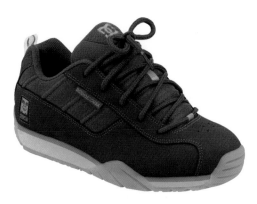

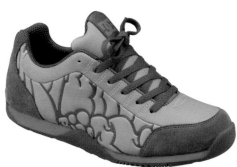

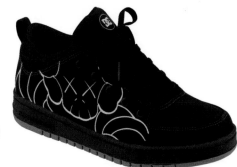

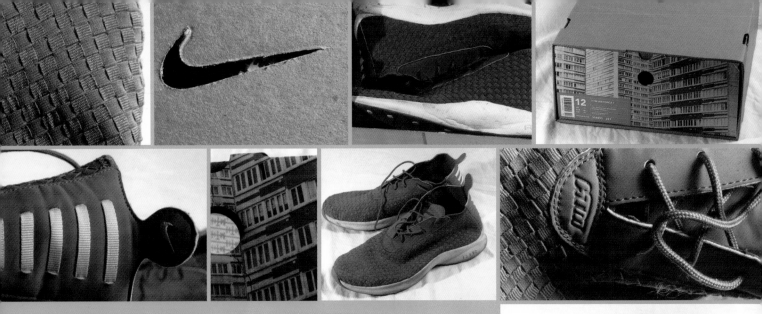

htm air woven

These 2002 releases are examples of Nike's collaboration with three designers. The H is for Japanese designer Hiroshi Fujiwara; the T is Nike's Jordan designer, Tinker Hatfield; and the M is for Mark Parker. The result is the HTM series of co-designed shoes. In this model, the group took the Woven design and simply made it into a boot cut with laces.

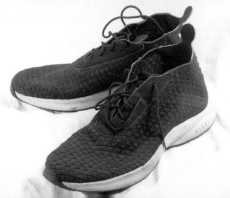

htm air force 1 lo

Released in 2002, this is another of the Nike/HTM (Hiroshi Fujiwara/Tinker Hatfield/Mark Parker) tripartite designer collaborations. In this case the group has reworked another classic from the Nike stable, the Air Force 1, with the niche and fashion markets firmly in mind.

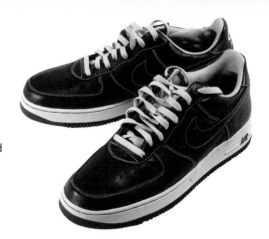

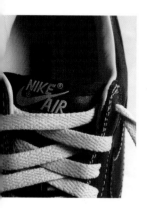
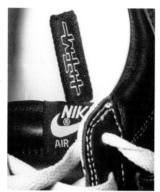
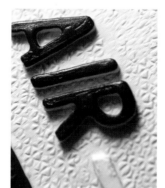
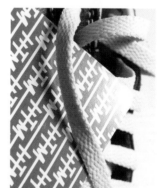
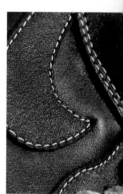

silas skate

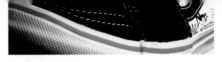

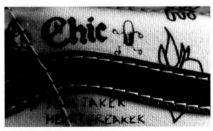

This is a recent Vans collaboration, which sees the brand working with the young fashion label Silas. Basically Vans allowed a few select design houses to come up with their own ideas for Vans skate shoes, thus putting Vans into a more fashion-orientated market. This version is a Silas graffiti-covered modern Skate Hi.

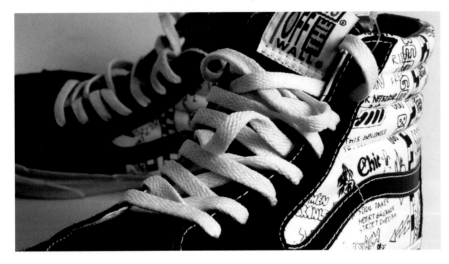

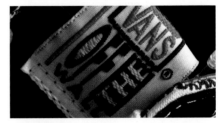

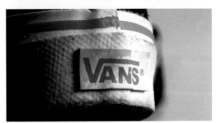

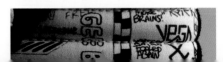

snoopy

It seems typical that Vans should be one of the first of the brands to work out that collaborations are a good thing. This Californian shoe company always took a liberal approach to its use of fabric, allowing customers to choose the material they wanted and then making the shoe up accordingly. This early collaboration with United Artists sees a Skate Hi Van covered in everybody's favourite hound, Snoopy.

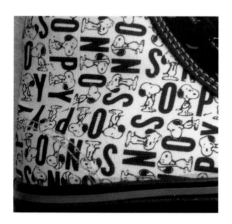

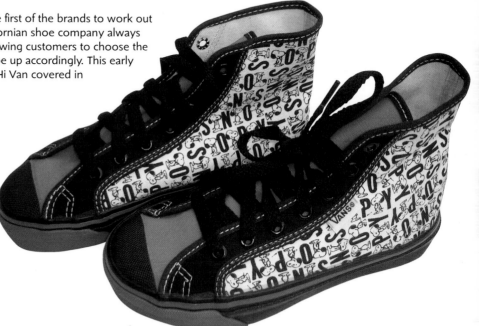

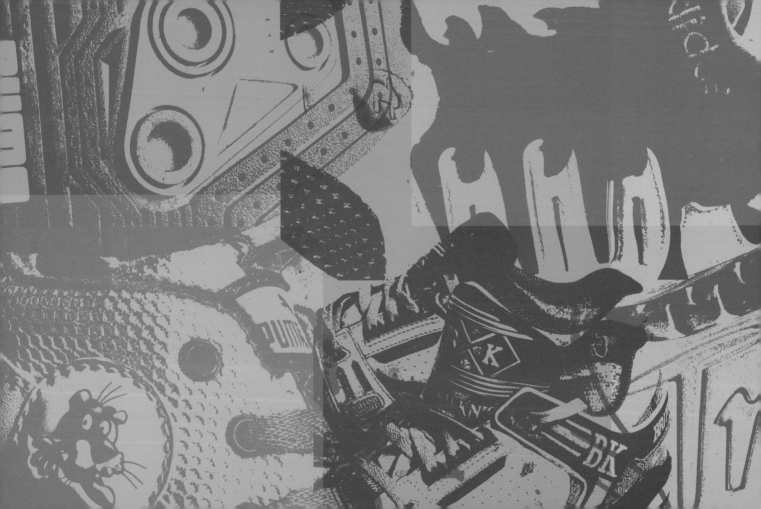

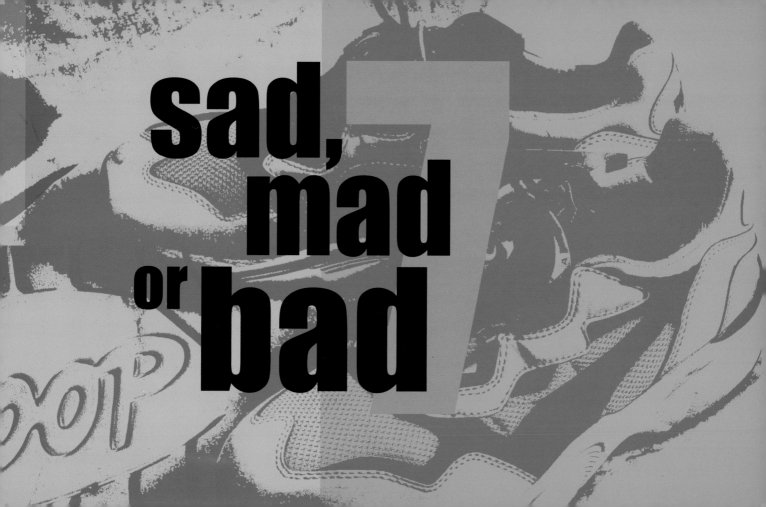

sad,
mad
or bad

sad, mad or bad
INTRODUCTION

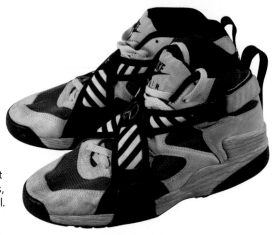

ABOVE Nike Air Raid Wood (*see page 376*).

One man's meat is another man's poison
or
Beauty is in the eye of the beholder

The trainer world is the same as any other walk of life, and what one person might like, another might well hate. The old clichés above sum this up perfectly. But regardless of whether you have an allegiance to a particular brand of trainers, whether you are an adi or a Nike fan, there are simply some shoes that cross all boundaries of allegiance or taste – these are the shoes that simply shock.

Some entrants in this chapter are not really 'bad' at all, but are more, well, 'mad'. That is the only way to sum them up. Others, however, for varying reasons are regarded more as being 'sad'. Perhaps they were attempts to jump on a particular style bandwagon in the hope of acquiring a degree of 'coolness'. Whatever the reason, they just didn't make it.

So inclusion in this chapter does not have to carry negative connotations, shoes here aren't necessarily dreadful. They have been included more for the fact that they elicit some unique response or cross the boundaries of eccentricity or taste. The line between innovative genius and utter nonsense can be hard to discern at times; sometimes something works and is truly fantastic, sometimes it simply misses the mark.

This, however, does not excuse everything. There are some shoes that no amount of hype or spin can justify. One entrant in the purely bad/sad category cannot be illustrated – nobody would admit to owning a pair. These are the L.A. Gear Billie Jeans designed by Michael Jackson from the 1980s, and the shoes came with metal straps and studs to match Michael's outfit from his Billie Jean album. Mind you, British Knights to some people's eyes, are another worthy inclusion in this chapter.

Anyway, take a look at the following shoes and make up your own mind.

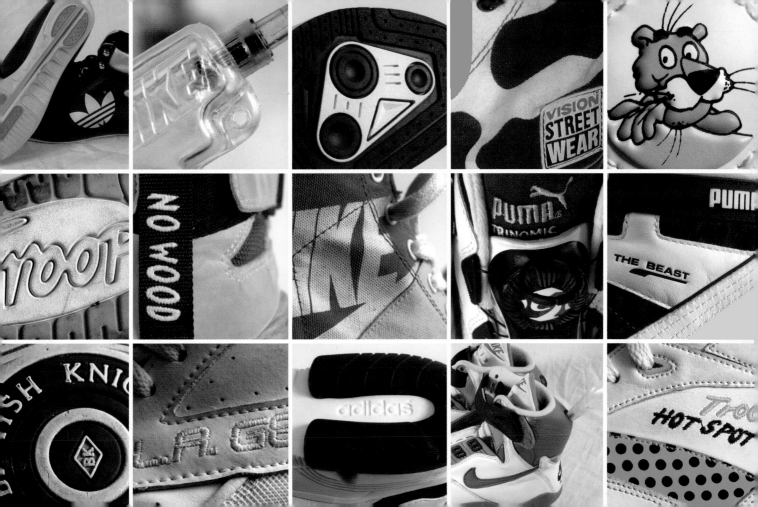

adidas ski boot

Officially called the Cross Country Ski, this shoe is an example of how adidas started to diversify, broadening its sporting expertise to include shoes suitable for all manner of sporting activities. Note, however, the huge adidas trefoil allied to the garish silver – although of questionable taste these are the hallmarks of a self-assured and confident brand.

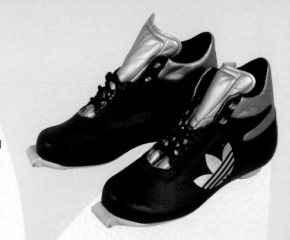

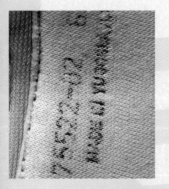

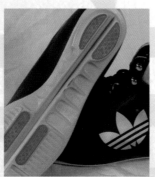

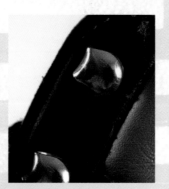

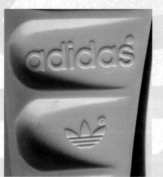

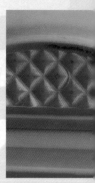

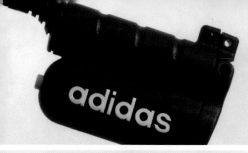
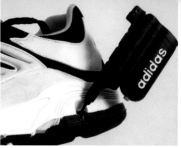
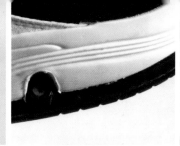
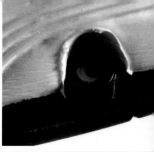
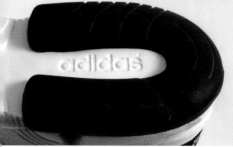
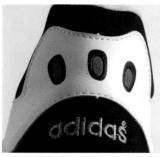
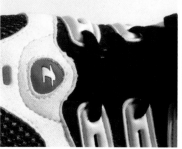
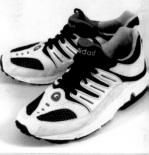
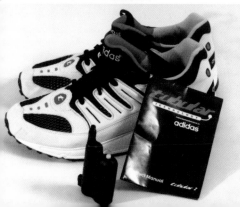

adidas tubular

The adidas Tubular, released in 1995, is an example of the struggle by the shoe brands trying to perfect an 'instant-pumping' system. Aesthetically poor, as you can see, the shoe was never popular. However, new technology made the pumping system more manageable and the air unit around the sole of the shoes was like walking on air.

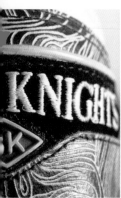
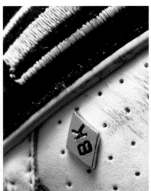
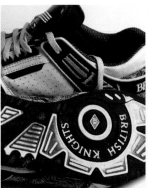
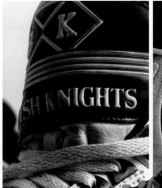
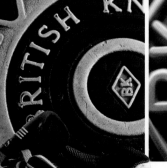

british knights

Once seen never forgotten. British Knights raised their head in the 1980s when many brands saw an opportunity to enter a new leisure-orientated trainer market. With no sporting heritage behind them, they relied on 'dubious' celebrity endorsees to enter the market. Fortunately, the trend ended as quickly as it started and British Knights are nowhere to be seen today.

L. A. gear

L.A. Gear, famous for developing shoes with a flashing sole (L.A. Lights) was a product of the 1980s trainer boom. In this same decade Reebok started a revolution, with its Freestyle gaining substantial sales growth. L.A. Gear came from nowhere to enter this lucrative market; with no sporting heritage it basically issued clones, such as this freestyle look-a-like. Sadly, it worked, but when Michael Jackson came on board with his Billie Jean range, it was a step too far. L.A. Gear went from nothing to the third top spot and back to nothing again in the space of a decade. Good riddance.

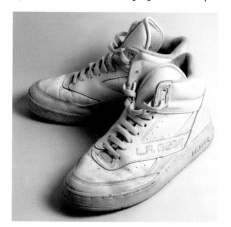
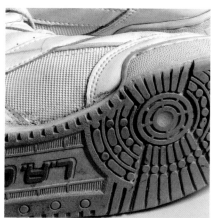
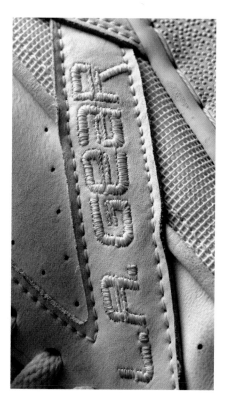

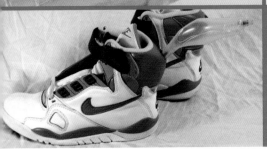

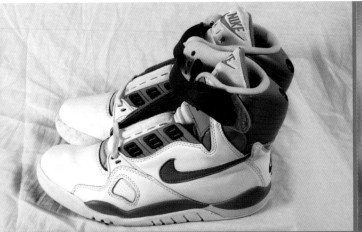

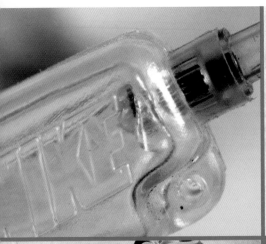

nike air pressure

The Air Pressure was released in 1989 and Nike hoped it would be the best basketball shoe available. It only came in one colourway, but innovative as it was, the system, with its own pump, and air valve inlet, never really worked. Nike designer Tinker Hatfield created the shoes worn by Marty McFly in *Back to the Future* from this model.

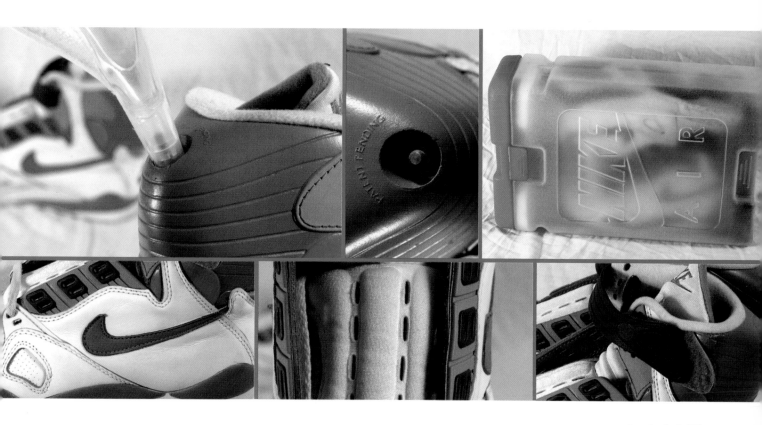

nike air raid wood

Nike released the Air Raid series in 1992, but this version was a homage to the basketball court. The shoe was designed for outdoor concrete surfaces, but as a nod to the old wooden courts, Nike put a wood-effect finish on top of the normal rubber sole unit. And to add insult to injury, a multicoloured peace sign was added to the cross strap.

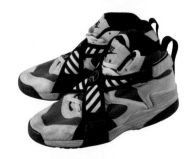

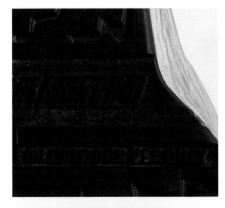

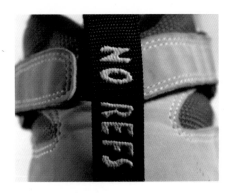

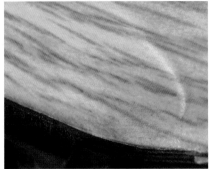

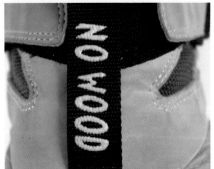

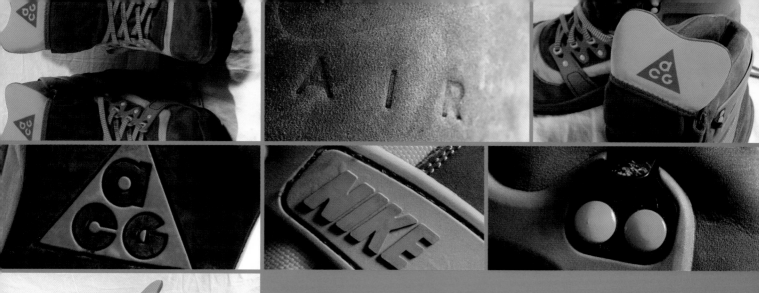

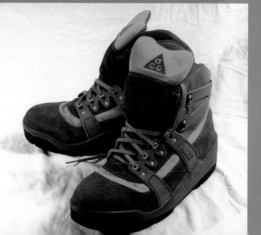

nike air super dome

The Air Super Dome was released in 1990 and was the highest specified of the walking shoes developed by Nike in the ACG (All Condition Gear) range. The Air Super Dome was designed with mountaineering and snow particularly in mind, and the model was derived from the earlier Lava Dome. However, rather than hiding the new shoe away due to its bulk, Nike decided to utilize super-loud colouring instead, in order to attain visibility in snow-covered terrain.

nike outbreak

Released in 1988, the Outbreak was Nike's initial attempt to enter the skateboarding market. This version is in canvas (it also came in leather) and it has the bold 'Big Nike' styling reminiscent of the era, but up the side of the shoe rather than on the heel. Popular response to these rare shoes gains them an entry in this chapter.

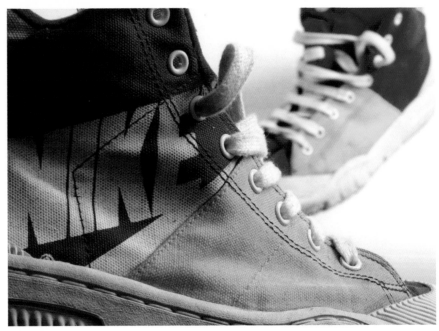

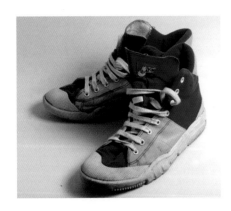

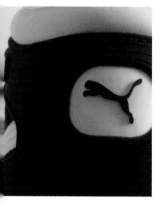
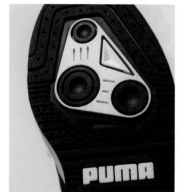
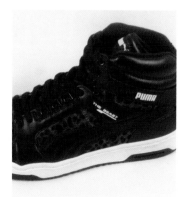
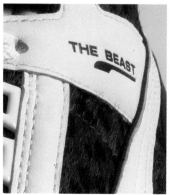
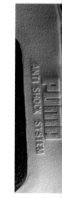

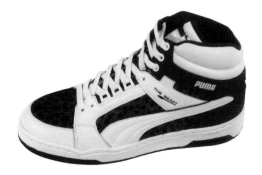

puma the beast

The Beast is an early 1980s' basketball shoe released in both hi and lo versions. But it's not for these facts that the Beast will be remembered. Now there is a proliferation of shoes made with fake materials, but in its day there were no other shoes made from fake leopardskin. Imagine it – the 1980s and its a furry trainer. Daring and brilliant.

puma pink panther

This model, released in the mid 1980s, is an example of collaboration between an established trainer brand and a commercial organization completely outside of the sporting arena. The Pink Panther speaks for itself, the 'Rinky Dink Panther' was a Panther that was positively Pink and well deserves its place here.

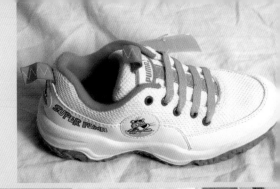

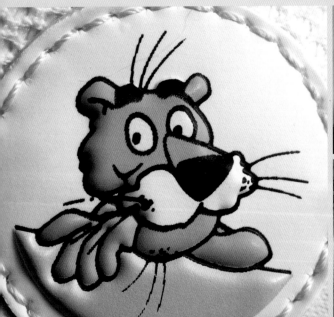

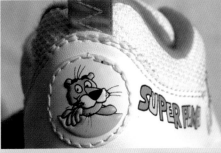

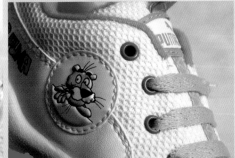

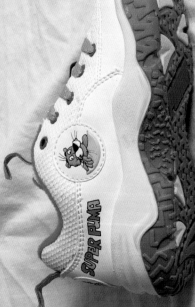

puma trinomic

Here is another example of the search for the laceless training shoe. Puma released the Trinomic system with a great fanfare in the 1990s. Actually the system did work, being a basic 'disk' system – when you twisted the disk it tightened the shoe, and all without laces. Despite this technological success the shoe never did particularly well and the system was soon dropped.

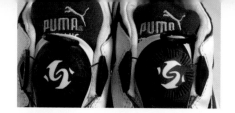

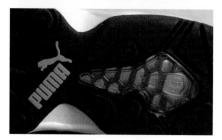

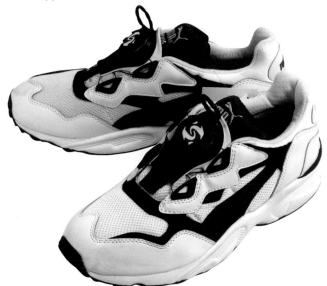

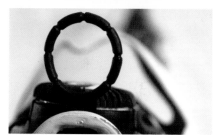

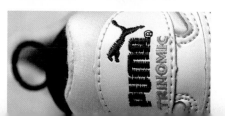

troop hot spot

The Troop Hot Spot is yet another entrant from the decade of bad taste. Troop was one of the brands that jumped on the bandwagon in the burgeoning and profitable trainer market of the 1980s. Like L.A. Gear, Troop paid particular attention to the aerobics exercise market, and this shoe is essentially a Reebok Freestyle derivative. Troop utilized non-sporting endorsees and fluorescent colours, as you can see, to attract a ladies' leisure market. This strategy worked for a while and then its time passed.

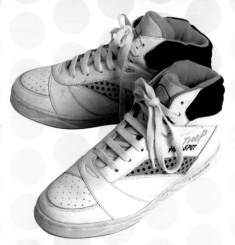

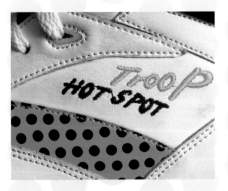

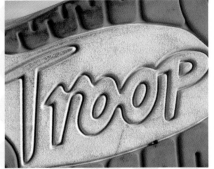

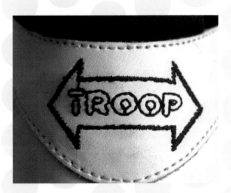

vision the moo

Vision was a skate shoe brand developed
by skateboarders for skateboarders and it
released its Vision Street Wear shoes in
the late 1980s. The shoes incorporated
skate features such as 'ollie pads', but the
Moo enters this section due to its mad
cowhide pattern. Vision wanted designs
that were rebellious and 'anti-hippie', and
which would give skaters a 'look' of
their own. The Moo
certainly did that.

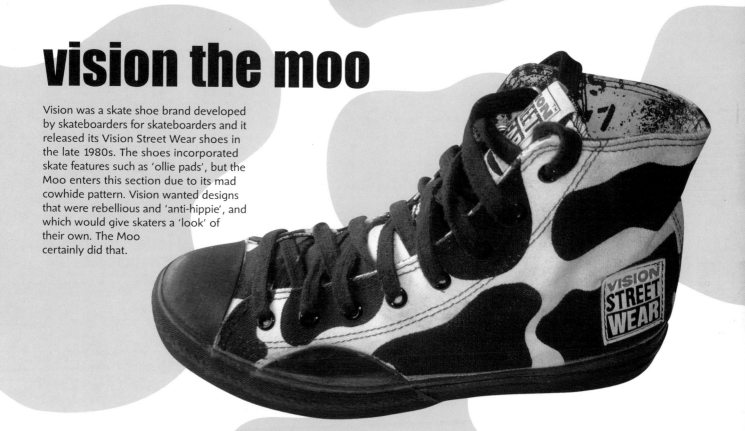

back to the future

back to the future

INTRODUCTION

It was the American author and philosopher Mark Twain who once remarked, 'History does not repeat itself, it just often rhymes'. Although his prophetic remark was certainly not uttered with trainers in mind, the quotation seems particularly relevant to today's scene.

Since the first edition of this book flew off the shelves, the whole world of trainers has exploded. It seems a month cannot pass without one of the giants or a new upstart company releasing a raft of new models upon an expectant public. It is the release or re-working of these models that brings the Twain quote to mind. The vast majority of new releases are re-issues, special customizations or new interpretations of old classics by some groovy young company or designer. It seems as if everybody has now collaborated with one of the 'established' firms to produce their own version of a classic model from the back catalogue.

This in itself is not a bad thing; some of the 're-interpretations' or collaborations are superb and add a new dimension to an old classic that makes the updated version even more contemporary or unique. However, for every good new design there is an equally poor example, and the phrase 'everything in moderation' springs to mind.

Gone are the days when it was only the established sporting brands that produced trainers. Now it seems every clothing or fashion firm makes them, too. Take a look at the various offerings from your once work-a-day local high-street shop: a small proportion are innovative, but most are just blatant rip-offs. Among the chaff are some gems. And it is in the hands of firms such as VisVim from Japan or the U.K.'s Duffer of St George that one day a huge trainer behemoth may arise.

Whatever happens, we can safely assume that the creativity is not going to stop and who knows where trainer designs will go next – so kick back and enjoy the trip.

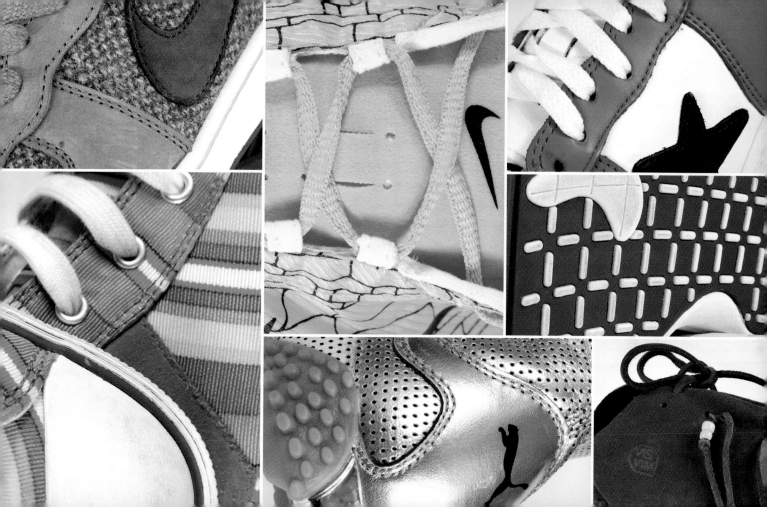

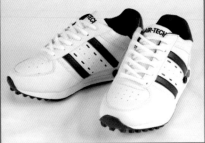

attack of the clones

AIR-TECH AND OTHERS

You must have seen some of these. 'Clone shoes' can be seen in many a street market or cheap shop near you. These trainers simply 'rip off' established brands, and this bastardized version exhibits the 'peg cushioning' and side stripes à la adidas, allied to a model name, Air-Tech, lifted from a 1980s range of Nikes.

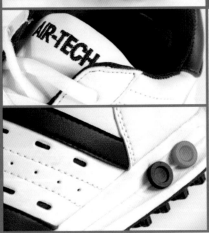

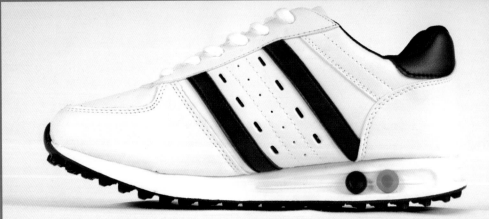

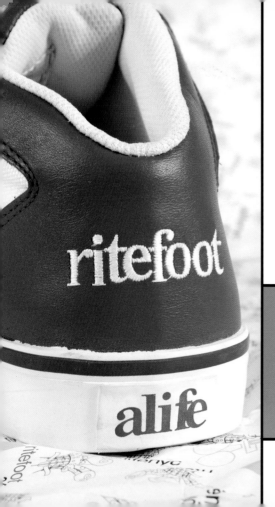

alife
UPTOWN

The trail-blazing of this brash new player on the scene is enjoyable to observe. The New York-based trainer collective Alife were one of the first to attempt to break into the monopoly of the 'big players'. Although sometimes producing models a little too reminiscent of previous offerings from other brands' stables, when they're on form Alife brings a breath of fresh air to a stale trainer world, while also opening doors for others to rush into.

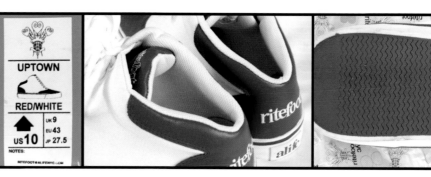

UPTOWN

RED/WHITE

	UK 9
	EU 43
US 10	JP 27.5

NOTES:

RITEFOOT@ALIFENYC.COM

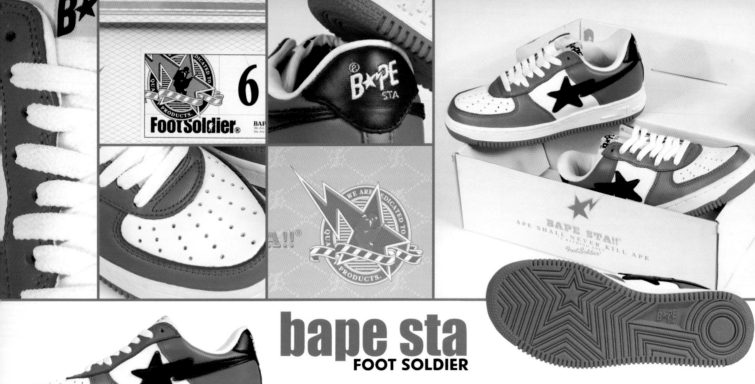

bape sta
FOOT SOLDIER

'Hipper than thou' Japanese clothing firm, A Bathing Ape, are now firmly established in trainer production, with a growing fan base slavishly following every move of head designer Nigo. To be honest, although very well made, these shoes are basically Air Force 1s with various tweaks and logos to give them that extra must-have feel.

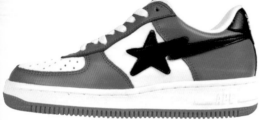

duffer

YOGI

If any 'new' brand should succeed, this is it. These boys were at the forefront of sourcing deadstock trainers when the idea was not even on the radar for most. The London-based clothing brand have entered a market they know a great deal about and their contributions, such as this Yogi, are rightly admired.

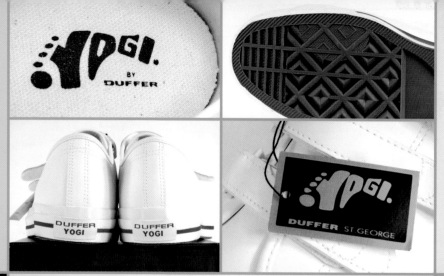

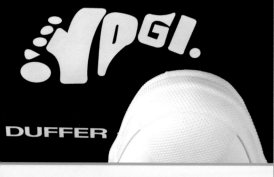

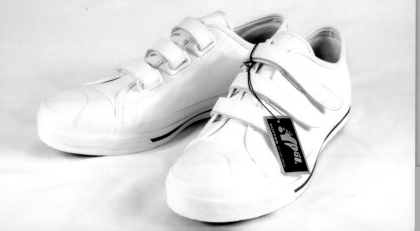

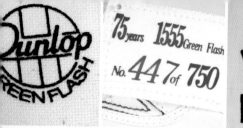

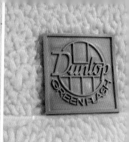

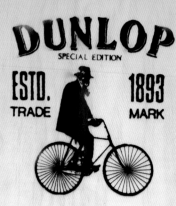

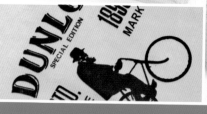

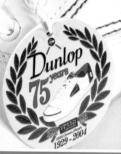

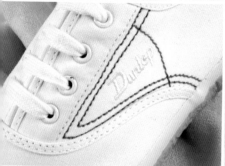

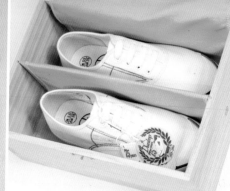

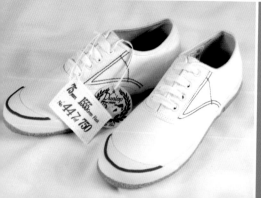

dunlop

GREENFLASH 75TH ANNIVERSARY

The old stalwart Dunlop brand have celebrated the 75th Anniversary of the Green Flash trainer, in production from 1929 to 2004. To commemorate the momentous occasion, Dunlop have re-launched a limited edition original design of the lace-up canvas trainer. All trainers are numbered 1 to 750, which is seen on the label.

dunlop

NAVY FLASH
CUSTOMIZED

Here Dunlop have modernized the classic Navy Flash. Using the maxim 'Dunlop is my Canvas', designer Adam Duffy has taken inspiration from the street and graffiti artists by utilizing a stencil method with bold retro designs including, 'Flash Is Back' and 'Drop Pants Not Bombs'.

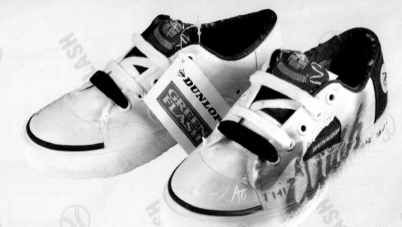

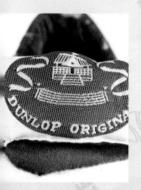

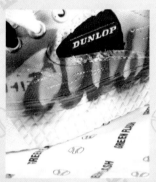

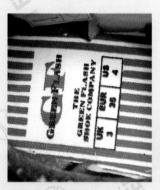

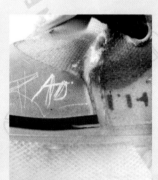

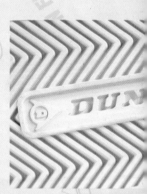

ENGINEERED TO
LAST FOR 100km
OF RUNNING   100km

ATTENTION: CONSTRUIT POUR
COURIR 100kms MAXIMUM

MAYFLY

>100 KM

nikebowerman.com

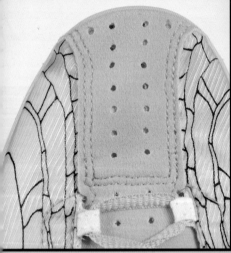

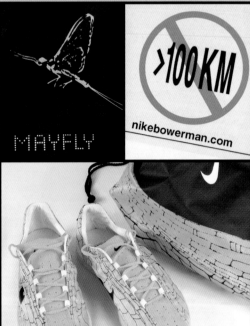

nike
MAYFLY

Nike co-founder Bill Bowerman believed the ultimate runner would support you just one meter past the finish line before wearing away. Apparently every extra 100g (3½ oz) you carry on your feet uses approximately 1% more energy to perform at the same level. So the Mayfly is lightweight and engineered to last for 100km (62 miles) of running/racing. Hence the name: the mayfly is an insect that lives, breeds and dies all in one day.

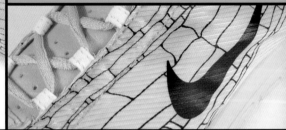

BOWERMAN

series

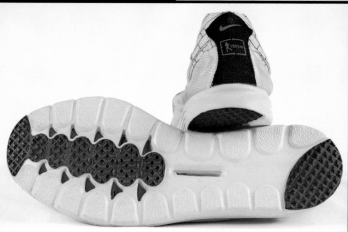

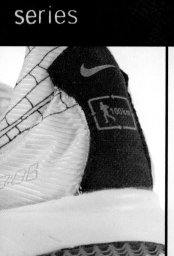

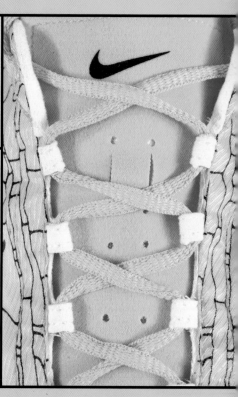

REUSE A MAYFLY
c/o NIKE RUNNING FOOTWEAR TEAM
EC-2A
NIKE EUROPE
COLOSSEUM 1
1213 NL HILVERSUM
THE NETHERLANDS

NIKE WILL RECYCLE THIS RACING SHOE IN ITS 'REUSE A SHOE' PROGRAM
IF YOU ARE KIND ENOUGH TO RETURN YOUR USED SHOES BACK TO US

NIKE VA RECYCLER CE MODELE DE COMPETITION DANS LE CADRE DE SON PROGRAMME
'RECYCLER UNE CHAUSSURE' SI VOUS NOUS RETOURNEZ VOTRE CHAUSSURE USEE - MERCI

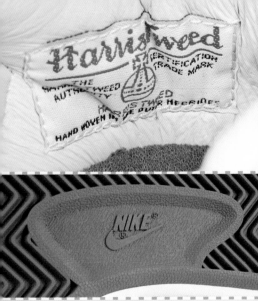

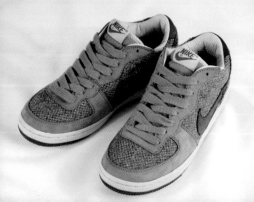

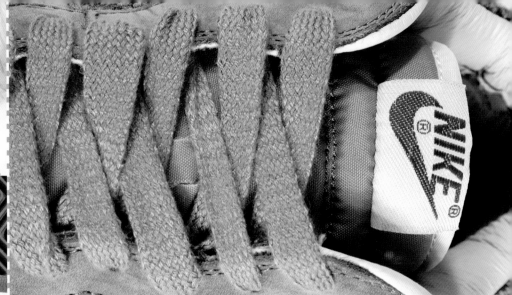

nike

HARRIS TWEED TERMINATOR

Definitely one of the more interesting re-workings of a classic model, Nike here juxtaposes the originally 'aggressive' Terminator from 1985 by softening it through utilizing the 'traditional' Harris Tweed fabric. Apparently it took 50 Scottish Hebridean Islanders to weave the quantity of fabric required for production.

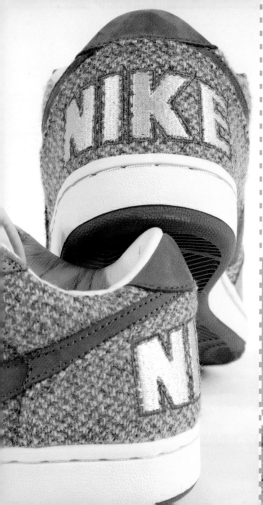

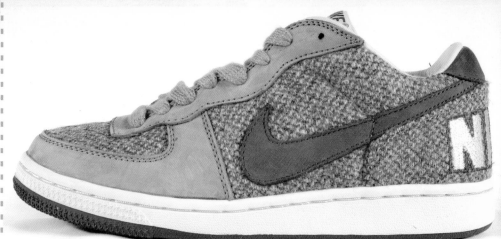

JUST DO IT

WMNS TERMINATOR LOW PRM TWD

7⁵

UK 5
EUR 38.5
CM 24.5

CLSC OLV / BAROQUE BRWN-BIRCH
OLIV / PLBRWN-BEIBOU

MADE IN VIETNAM / FABRIQUE AU VIETNAM
HECHO EN VIETNAM

309878 321   WWW.NIKE.COM

pony

SHOOTER

Although mainly known in their USA homeland, it's good to see one of the old faithfuls raising its profile again. Founded in 1972, Pony's heyday came in the 1980s, a period to which they seem forever linked. It is from this era that we see the re-release of the Shooter, one of their 'de ja viewed' collection, in which Pony re-introduces some of their classic models.

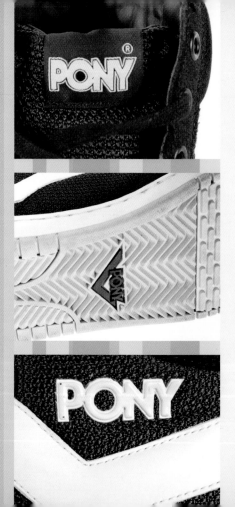

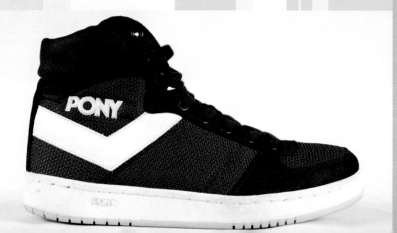

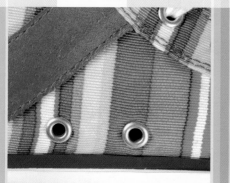

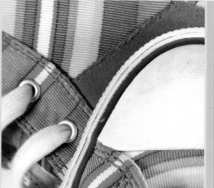

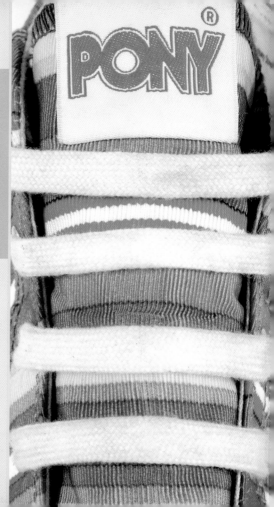

pony
UPTOWN

As well as releasing simple standards, Pony have re-worked old models in new bright and distinctive styles, like this radical multi-colouring of the classic canvas Uptown baseball boot, first released in 1978. The innovative update is reminiscent of Pony's original slogan, 'Pound the streets, reach for the skies'.

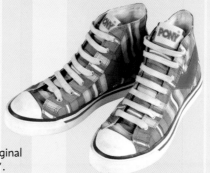

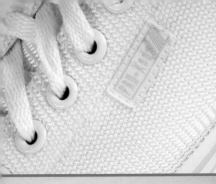

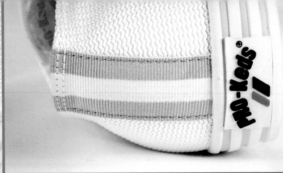

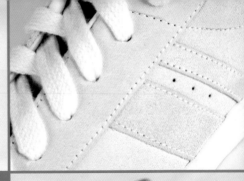

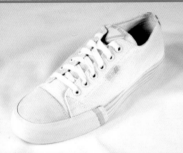

pro-keds

SUPER MESH, PISTOL PETE AND AVIATOR

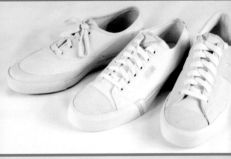

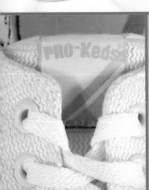

This original American brand have reached into their back catalogue to update and release new versions with the classic leisure market firmly in mind. The Pistol Pete version is named after an infamous 1970s basketball player while the Aviator is in honour of the Pro-Keds-wearing madcap billionaire Howard Hughes.

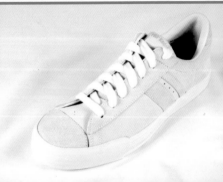

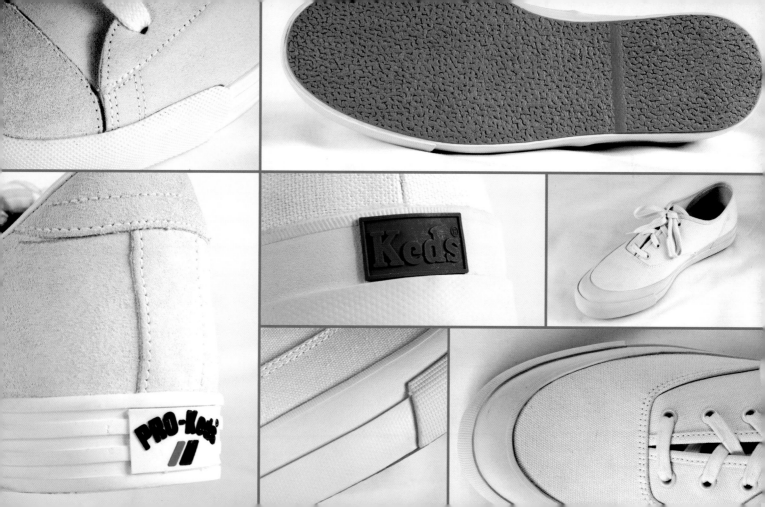

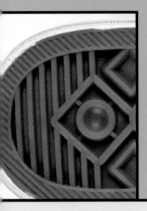
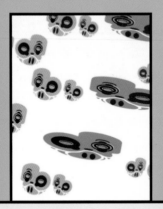
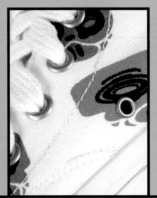
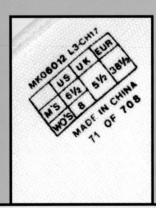
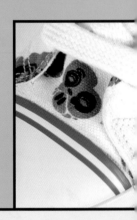

MK06012 L3-CH17

	US	UK	EUR
M'S	6½	6	
WO'S	8	5½	38½

MADE IN CHINA
71 OF 708

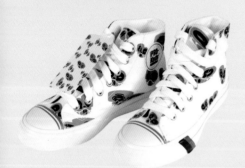

pro-keds

NYC LASE

Pro-Keds re-working of a classic model is part of the company's 'Artist Series', a limited edition re-working of various models with a selection of artists. NYC Lase was New York's first 'excessive aggressive' street bomber. His 'tag' would appear consecutively throughout the streets of New York. I bet he never thought one day he would be paid to 'vandalize' sneakers!?

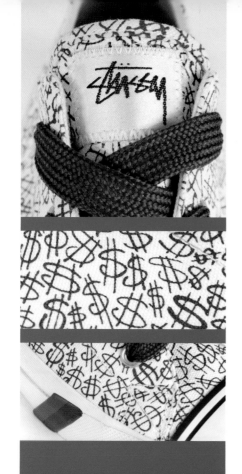

pro-keds
STUSSY

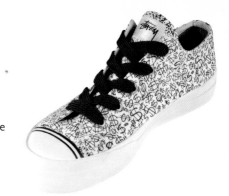

The final entry from Pro-Keds makes it a full house of trainer trends, with this re-working of an old-skool classic – the Royal Low. Given a new makeover by hip streetwear label Stussy, the shoe exhibits a graphic $$$ print to produce a new slant and modern feel.

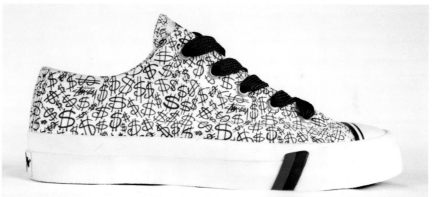

puma
PHILIPPE STARCK LOW

A particularly interesting slant on collaborations sees designer Philippe Starck, in an exclusive development with the Museum of Modern Art, develop the low version of his 'Evolutionary Shoe', a collaboration with Puma. The pared-down trainer resembles a clog, and logos are discreetly hidden on the back and bottom of the sneaker, which is grey and yellow with an orange interior.

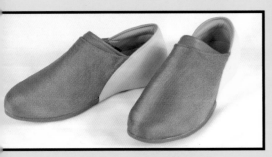

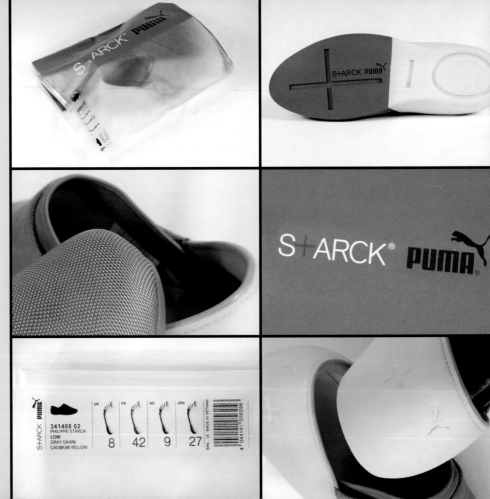

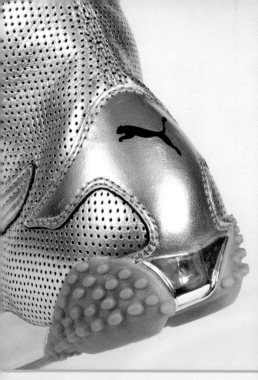

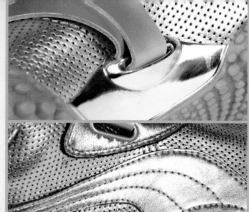

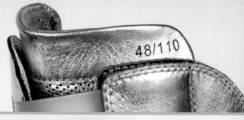

48/110

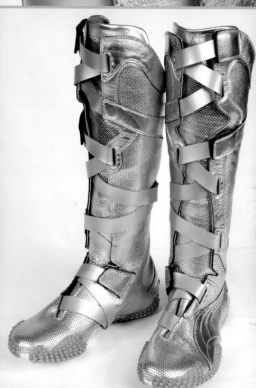

puma
MOSTRO ALTO BOOT

Considering the blurb, 'Bold, daring and avant-garde are just a few ways to describe the new Puma Mostro Alto boot', I would use one word, 'Mad'! Refreshingly alternative, the model is a boot version of Puma's modern cult classic Mostro trainer. As seen here, if you want to stand out that bit more, choose the limited edition gold metallic.

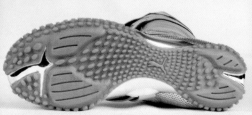

puma

SUEDE OLYMPIC EDITION

To celebrate what could be probably called their signature shoe, a special limited edition range of the legendary Puma Suede and Leather Basket has been introduced, offering four styles inspired by four different Olympic games – Munich, LA, Mexico and Tokyo. Each shoe has its own colourway, an Olympic flame stitched into the fabric of the shoe and features the year of the games they represent. Only a limited run of the shoes is available.

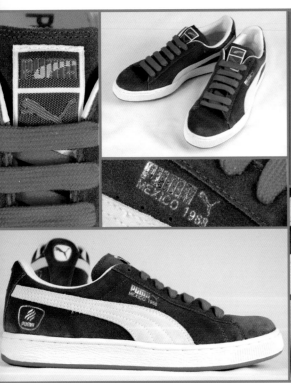

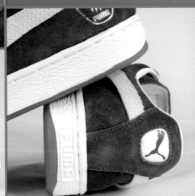

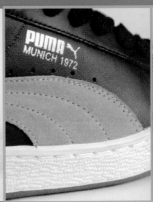

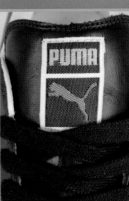

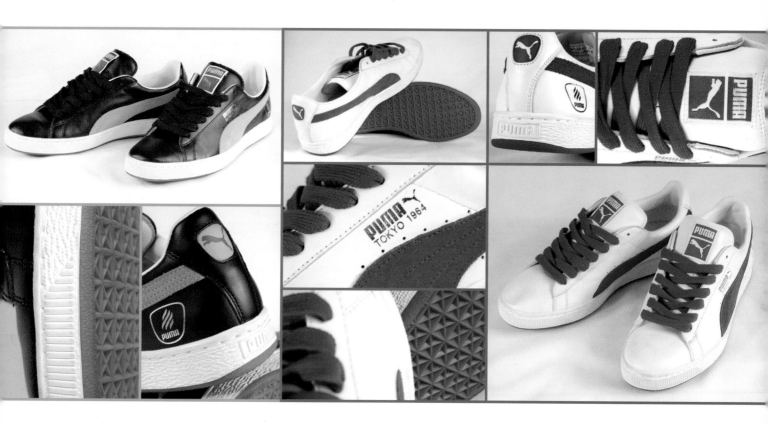

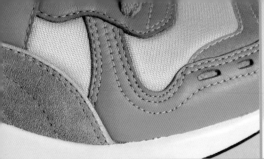

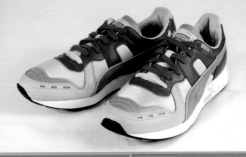

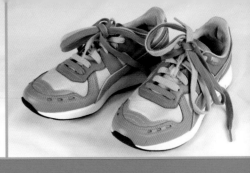

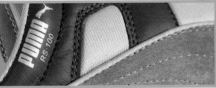

puma
RS-100

The RS-100 LE seen here is a modern release with a nod to Puma's past. The model was first introduced in 1986 as a Computer Shoe. The RS could be connected to a computer of the day via a cable and floppy disc provided. The new takedown version loses the now defunct computer but retains the look and feel of the original – only in vibrant colour combinations and two sets of laces.

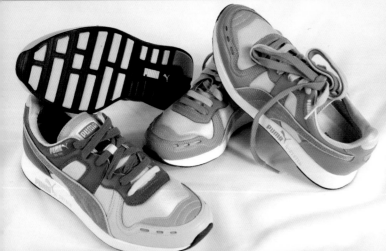

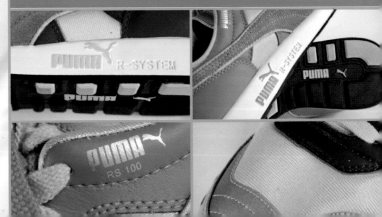

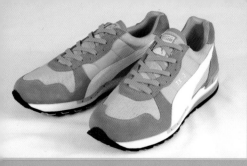

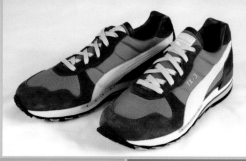

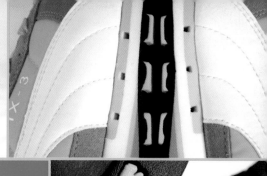

A re-working of a technological running classic, the TX3 which was first introduced in 1987, has been released as part of Puma's 'lifestyle' footwear range. In keeping with modern trainer trends, this range aims to fuse modern elements with traditional Puma style, offering a running shoe with a lifestyle twist, updated with some nice reflective details, and vibrant colourways, too.

puma
TX-3

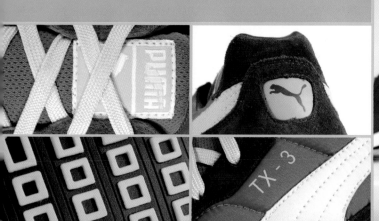

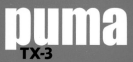

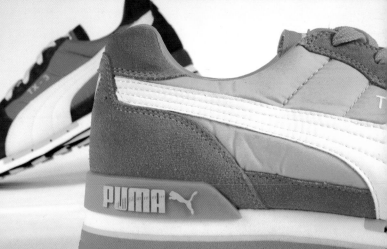

reebok
S. CARTER COLLECTION

Yet another example on the endless seam of collaborations, this trainer shows Reebok hooking up with S. Carter, better known as hiphop legend Jay-Z. Importantly it is aimed at the urban leisure market. The model is the first release in the collection by Rbk, and as the man himself says, 'People who check out the S. Carter Collection should know that this definitely meets my high standards and expectations.'

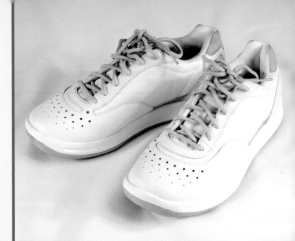

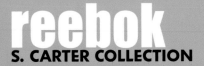

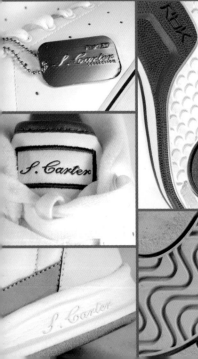

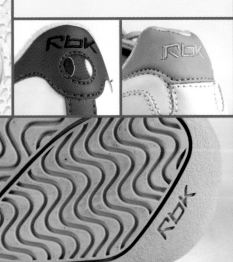

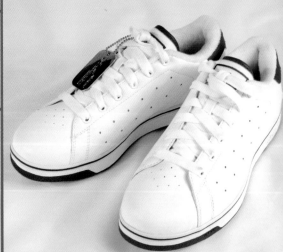

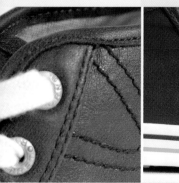
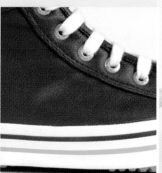
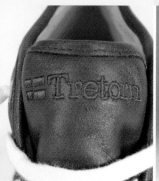
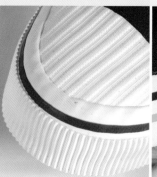
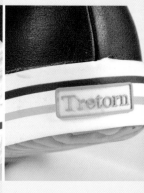

tretorn

GULLWING HOCKEY BOOT

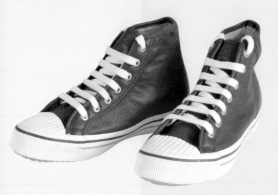

Long established in their own country but now garnering more of an international profile, Tretorn is one example of how the trainer world is getting bigger. However, this brand are not exactly newcomers. Sweden's Tretorn brand were established in 1891 and all their shoes were made in Helsinborgs until the mid 1980s. This hockey boot re-issue features the brands signature gullwing stitching.

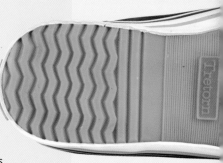

vans
ADDICT ERA

Exhibiting the current fashion of all things re-interpreted, old-skool skate brand Vans have opened their back catalogue for a re-working in their 'Vault' series. These Eras have been given a fresh feel through a collaboration with the British streetwear label, Addict. It uses the brand's 'A Monogram' pattern, which has a strong resemblance to the Vans checkerboard pattern, thus keeping a traditionalist vibe to the co-lab shoe.

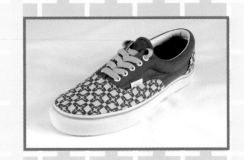

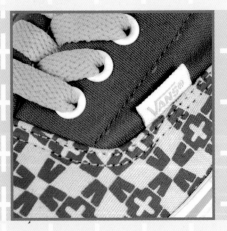

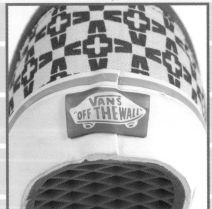

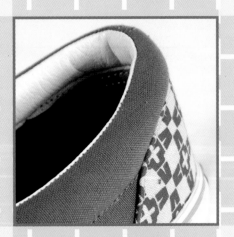

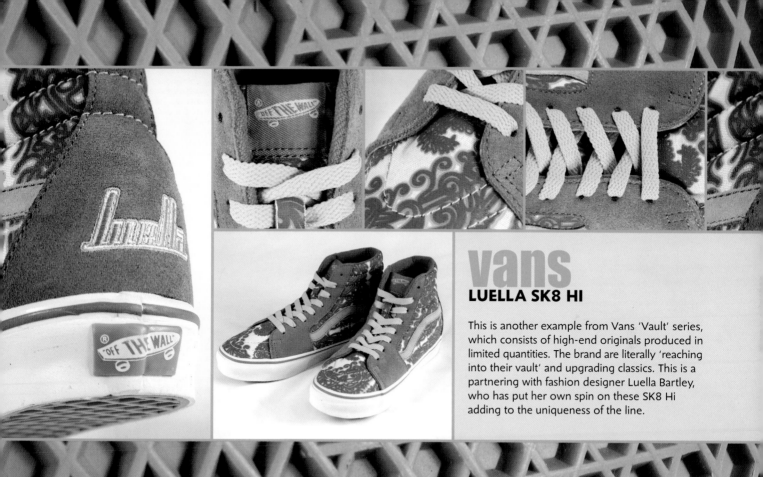

vans

LUELLA SK8 HI

This is another example from Vans 'Vault' series, which consists of high-end originals produced in limited quantities. The brand are literally 'reaching into their vault' and upgrading classics. This is a partnering with fashion designer Luella Bartley, who has put her own spin on these SK8 Hi adding to the uniqueness of the line.

vans
SLAYER

An interesting slant on the collaboration front sees Vans produce the Originals Collection. This is a programme of ongoing workings with bands and musicians who love Vans. Made to the exact specifications of the original skateboarding shoes, this version of the 'old-skool' model is by Metal band Slayer, while another is by Motorhead!

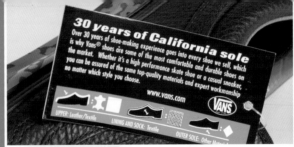

30 years of California sole
Over 30 years of shoe-making experience goes into every shoe we sell, which is why Vans® shoes are some of the most comfortable and durable shoes on the market. Whether it's a high performance skate shoe or a casual sneaker, you can be assured of the same top-quality materials and expert workmanship no matter which style you choose.

www.vans.com

UPPER: Leather/Textile   LINING AND SOCK: Textile   OUTER SOLE: Other Material

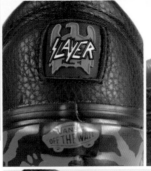

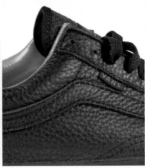

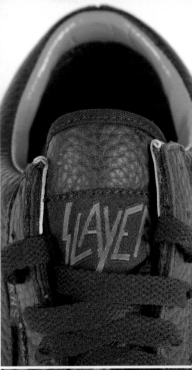

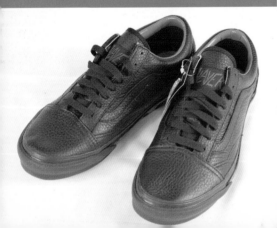

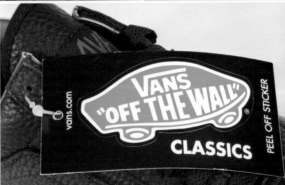

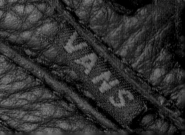

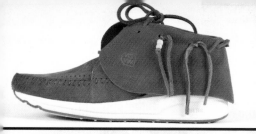

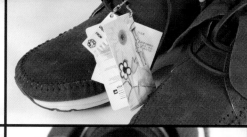

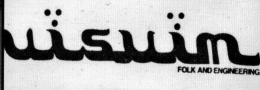

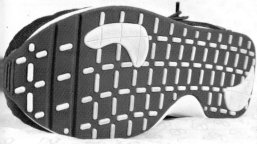

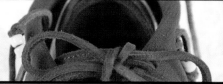

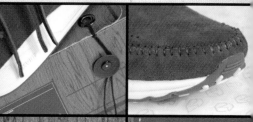

visvim

FBT

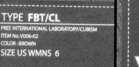

TYPE **FBT/CL**
FREE INTERNATIONAL LABORATORY/CUBISM
ITEM No. V006-02
COLOR : BROWN
SIZE US WMNS 6

visvim.
MADE IN KOREA / FABRIQUE EN KOREA / HECHO EN KOREA

In my humble opinion, this is simply the best new shoe designed in the last few years. To boot, it's from a small Japanese brand set up by Hiroki Nakamura in 2001. The inspiration for the shoe comes from an album cover of the band 'Fun Boy Three' (hence the name FBT), featuring the band's singer and founder Terry Hall wearing a pair of Ska boy's '80s moccasins.

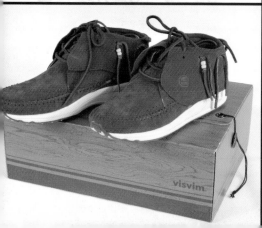

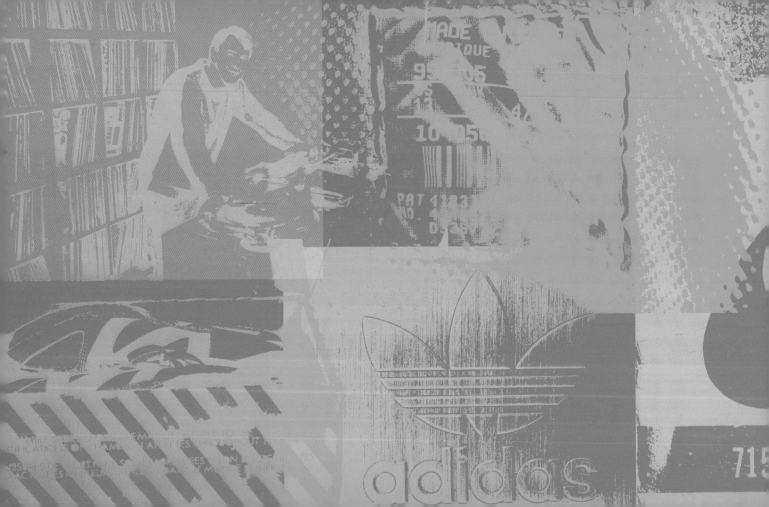

9

collecting

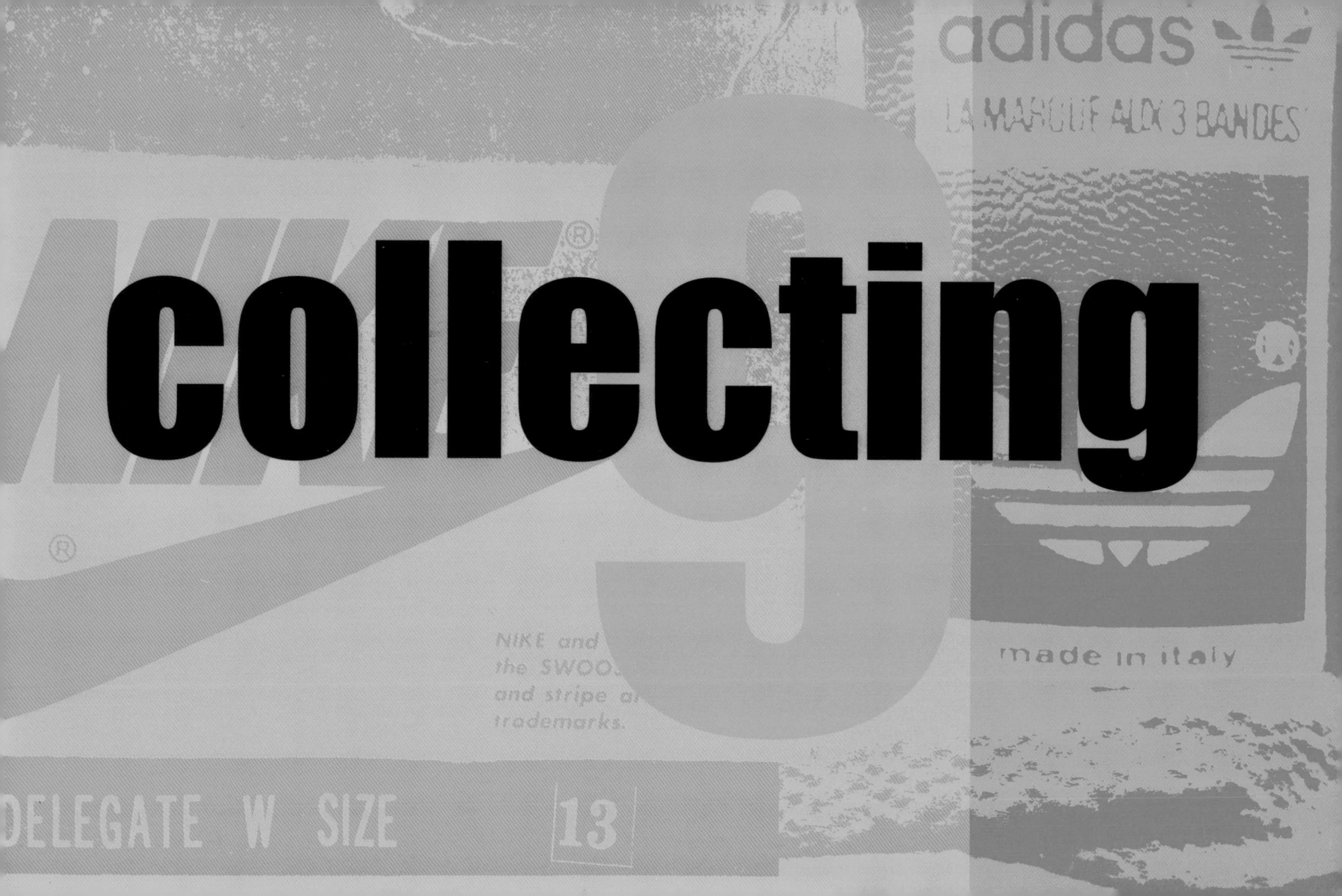

collecting

INTRODUCTION

Trainers are not only collected as practical, aesthetically pleasing items of footwear, they can also represent a connection with the past – it's not unusual, for people to recall events by associating them with the trainers they were wearing at the time. But many people own numerous pairs of trainers but don't think of themselves as collectors. For them, it's as simple as seeing a pair of trainers, liking them and buying them.

Whatever your reason for buying trainers – whether you want to wear them, store them or sell them – there are a few basic rules to follow. Trainers are always worth substantially more in their original box, and it goes without saying that the better the condition, the more you have to pay. Once you get involved with collecting, you will come across the term 'deadstock'. These are trainers that are boxed and pristine but have never been worn and are always worth looking for. Shoe size also has an effect on value – for example, in the U.K. sizes 8–11 (in the U.S. sizes 9–12) are most desirable because these are the popular shoe sizes.

Original issue shoes have a higher value. Once a model has been made and released it can sometimes be released again at a later date. These later releases are called re-issues and are always less valuable. And there are certain models that are more collectable than others. These, however, vary over time as fashion and preferences change, but probably the most collected shoes are those in the Nike Jordan series. Bear in mind that a trainer does not have to be old to be collectable – certain issues, either limited or 'hyped', become instantly desirable. Watch for trainers with composite soles, which were common in the late 1970s and 1980s, as these soles degrade even if the shoes have never been worn. If you can, bend a shoe; if it is weak the sole will show signs of cracking.

If, like me, you wear all your trainers, then cleaning is sometimes necessary. Here is a basic cleaning and care list:

1 It is always best to hand wash trainers using warm water and a brush to avoid shrinkage or damage.
2 Keep trainers out of direct sunlight to prevent fading.
3 Serious collectors keep their shoes in airtight containers to limit degradation.

Collecting should not just be about value. Although rare items will always be sought after, get involved with collecting only if you have a genuine love for the object or commodity. Anyway, whatever your reasons, this chapter details a few tips to help you find that special shoe.

collector
FRASER MOSS

Back in the late 1980s a very select group of trainer 'archaeologists' recognized the demand for models of trainers that were no longer in production. One of these, YMC's Fraser Moss, allied his love of sports shoes with an entrepreneurial spirit to source deadstock classics.

NH: How did it all begin?

FM: Well it was two things. I have always loved trainers, I worked in a sports store as my first job, and I have always had a collector's mentality – from comic books to records. I knew that certain things were guaranteed to be collectable at some point in the future.

NH: So you jumped in and started sourcing deadstocks?

FM: Well back in about 1989 there was one guy, Trevor Norris, who owned a shop called Utopia, and he was importing deadstock from America. At that time he was selling it for less than you'd pay for a new pair of trainers, even though these were original boxed Puma States or adidas shell-toes! People wanted it, but there was no collector's market as there is now. So people like me started buying it up.

NH: Which particular finds stick in your mind?

FM: One find I remember was in Ron Jones Sports of Maesteg. After initial persuasion Ron let us go into his stockroom – the Holy Grail for deadstock hunters. We'd been buying up his old deadstock for months, but we hadn't even looked at what he was selling in the store. And there they were – a whole size break of Jordan 1s, boxed and perfect. We shipped them to Japan and sold them for 20 times what we paid.

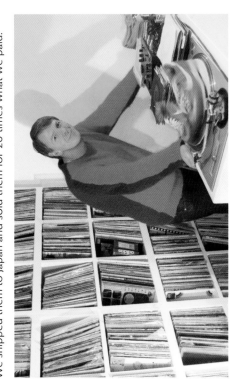

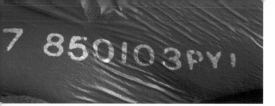

7 850103PY1

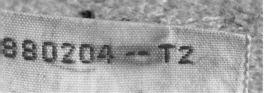

880204 — T2

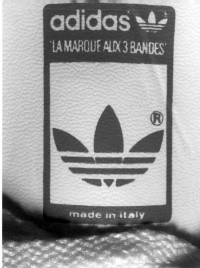

NIKE TIPS You can date Nikes by the code inside the shoes: The first two digits of the code give you the year the shoes were made – in the examples here (*above*), 1985 and 1988. The label (*below*) gives a date for these shoes of 1995.

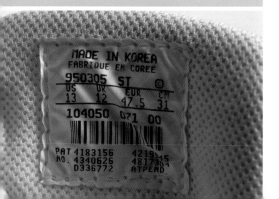

MADE IN KOREA
FABRIQUE EM COREE
950305 ST ©
US   UK   EUR   CM
13   12   47.5   31
104050 071 00

PAT 4183156   4219545
NO. 4340626   4817364
   D336772   ATPEND

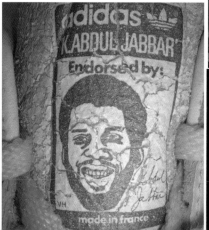

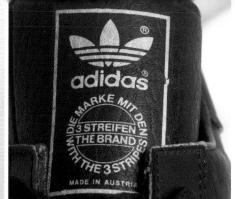

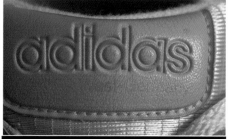

ADIDAS TIPS One way to tell if adidas shoes are old originals (therefore collectable) is from the tongue. The older models were most often made in Europe, so look out for labels 'made in' France, Italy, West Germany, Yugoslavia and Austria.

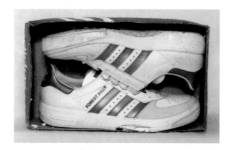

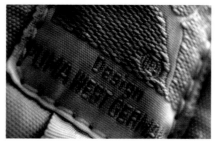

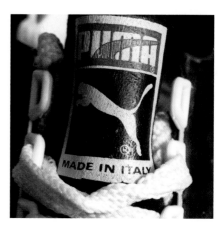

OTHER TIPS On older shoes, especially those made from compound rubber (*above left*), watch out for deteriorating sole units. When buying, bend them if possible – if they are weak, they will crack. Adidas were not the only ones that used to make their shoes in Europe; it is also a way to identify original Pumas, like these from Italy and West Germany (*above middle and right*).

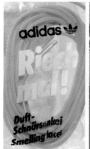

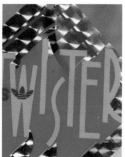

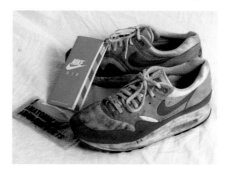

ACCESSORIES The market in rare and deadstock trainers has grown even bigger since the advent of internet auction sites, such as e-bay. Bear in mind that values will increase dramatically (and authenticity will be easier to verify) if the shoes come with their original 'extras'. Always try and keep (or look out for) such accessories as laces, labels, shoe insteps and booklets, as illustrated here (*left*). Try and keep these in good condition as well in order to maximize value.

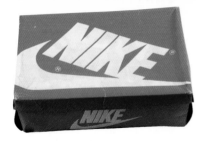

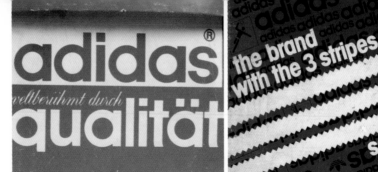

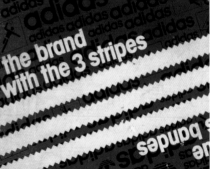

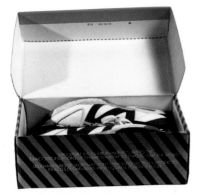

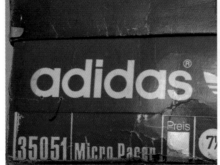

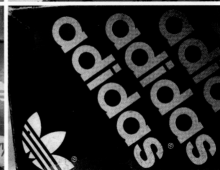

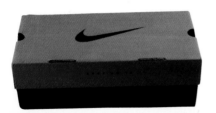

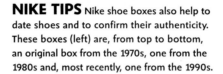

NIKE TIPS Nike shoe boxes also help to date shoes and to confirm their authenticity. These boxes (left) are, from top to bottom, an original box from the 1970s, one from the 1980s and, most recently, one from the 1990s.

ADIDAS TIPS Like Nike, adidas have altered their box design over the years. For authenticity and maximum value, any shoe should come with its original box. Look for the old trefoil logo, original model names and older branding on boxes.

BOXES AND PACKAGING Trainers are more collectable and valuable if they come in as near to new condition as possible. If trainers come with their original packaging then authenticity is more assured and the shoes' value to collectors increases. Shown here, from left to right, are examples of an older-style Puma box, an extremely rare Nike waffle-soled sandals box with a portrait of Bill Bowerman on the lid, the original and highly unusual plastic box for the Nike Air Pressure shoes and finally an original P-F Flyers hinged-lid box.

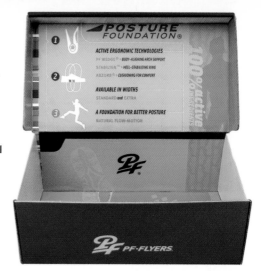

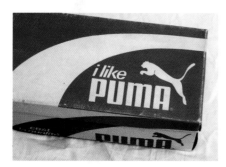

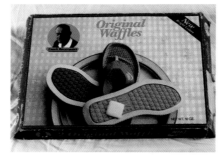

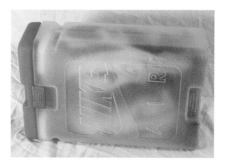

importer
ROBERT WADE SMITH

Robert Wade Smith's pioneering Liverpool shop was the first of its kind in the U.K. Earlier in his career, in the late 1970s, he was controller of 25 adidas concessions across the country and it was at this point he noticed the city of Liverpool's desire for the brand with the three stripes.

Seeing obvious potential growth in the market, Wade Smith was keen to sell more varied stock in Liverpool. Unfortunately, this view was not shared by adidas management, who thought that the high sales figures were merely a passing fad. History was to prove Wade Smith's instincts correct and massive sales in Liverpool leading up to Christmas 1980 convinced him that he now wanted his own store.

Getting adidas on side was crucial for his planned new venture – if adidas refused to provide stock for him, for example, he'd be in trouble. Going straight to the top, Wade Smith pitched his idea and won the support of chairman Thomas Black. Unfortunately, adidas U.K. management was not happy. He was frozen out, lost his position as controller, given a representative job instead, and, some months later, was made redundant. This was just the incentive he needed. Travelling to

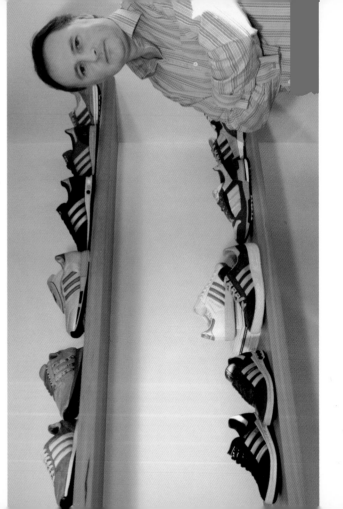

Liverpool, Wade Smith found a backstreet store, fitted it out, and bought the shoes he needed. Unfortunately, on the morning of his grand opening, he arrived to discover that thieves had broken in and stolen 70 per cent of his entire stock.

Well, when something like that happens right at the beginning of a venture, things can only get better. Trading with his remaining stock he noticed a steady flow of soccer fans in the store wearing adidas Trimm Trabs. Asking where they were buying their trainers, the standard answer was always Brussels, which he presumed they were travelling through en route to their teams' away matches in Europe.

Shutting the store in its second week, our budding businessman made his way to Brussels with a few empty suitcases, only to find nothing there. He bought up a few pairs of Pumas (they wouldn't supply him at the time), but it was adidas he was really after. Before boarding the ferry on his way home, Wade Smith bumped into five lads all with Trimm Trabs or Grand Slams on their feet. Explaining that he'd just opened his store in Liverpool, he offered to take any trainers off their hands they'd bought on their travels. He'd struck lucky at last.

On the way home they showed him their haul – Trimm Trabs in different colours, as well as München and Grand Slam trainers. He offered to buy the lot and the next day, waiting for him when he opened his store, were the lads he'd met with bags full of trainers to sell him. Agreeing a price, Wade Smith bought 25 pairs and by the end of the day he'd sold them all except for two pairs. This was to be the most magical day in the store's history and indeed the beginning of a new era.

On the back of this success, Wade Smith hired a van and arranged with his bank to withdraw every penny of his available overdraft. He drove to London to collect the money in cash, and started out on a high-tension journey to Aachen (just outside of Cologne). His plan was to buy as many pairs of adidas as possible from the main dealer there. All in all, his money stretched to 475 pairs, and when the dealer asked him to come back the next day with a banker's draft, Wade Smith told him he would pay now – and in cash. Astonished (he'd never been made such a cash offer before for so many shoes in one day), the dealer gave him another five per cent discount on the spot.

After a couple of similar journeys to Germany in the following seven weeks he was on his way, supplying the insatiable appetite in Liverpool for rare trainer imports. Soon enough, he was importing shoes from Austria, Germany, France and Ireland. Although it is near impossible to repeat the buzz he created in Liverpool all those years ago, to this day the Wade Smith reputation has been built on selling rare products. The revolutionary attitude in the early 1980s saw Wade Smith create a following in Liverpool that continues strongly today.

SOURCES & SITES

WEBSITES

Independent Sites – Information, Chat and Sales

http://sneakers.pair.com
reference to models and manufacturers

www.chucksconnection.com
everything you need to know about the Converse Chuck Taylor

www.crookedtongues.com
reviews, features and shop

www.deadshoescrolls.com
nothing for sale but some interesting information

www.mrsneaker.com
imports for sale

www.pipcom.com/~tempus/sneakers/
information and trainer histories

www.snapsorama.com
deadstock vintage stock for sale

www.sneakerfan.com
specially for adidas fans. Includes interviews and reviews

www.sneakerfreaks.co.uk
deadstock vintage trainer sales and chat

www.sneakerking.de
vintage deadstock trainers for sale

www.sneaker-nation.com
the original trainer site, includes chat and information

www.sneakerpimp.com
rare and imported trainers and chat

www.terraceretro.com
all things football and trainers

Auction Sites

www.ebay.com
the biggest and best – if you want trainers, you can't beat it

www.vintageusa.com
the original vintage auction site, a good resource

Official Brand Sites

www.adidas.com
www.asics.com
www.asicstiger.com
www.bata.com
www.converse.com
www.dcshoecousa.com

www.diadora.com
www.etnies.com
www.fila.com
www.gola.co.uk
www.greenflash.co.uk
www.kswiss.com
www.newbalance.com
www.nike.com
www.pony.com
www.prokeds.com
www.puma.com
www.reebok.com
www.saucony.com
www.tsubo.com
www.vans.com

Shopping Sites

www.mytrainers.com
www.officeholdings.co.uk
www.soletrader.co.uk
www.footlocker.com
www.retrotredz.com
www.jdsports.co.uk
www.modells.com
www.retroshoestore.com

SHOPS

Alife Rivington Club
158 Rivington Street
New York, NY 10012
Tel: 212 375 8128

Arch 47 (What goes around
comes around)
The Stables Market
Chalk Farm Road
London NW1 8AH
Tel: 020 7388 3968

Footlocker U.K Ltd
(and shops worldwide)
191–209 Camden High Street
London NW1 7BT
Tel: 020 7482 6294

JD Sports Ltd
30–31 Kings Mall
King Street
London W6 0QB
Tel: 020 8748 8175

Meteor Sports
408–410 Bethnal
Green Road
London E2 0DJ
Tel: 020 7739 0707

My Trainers
9 Shorts Gardens
London WC2H 9AZ
Tel: 020 7379 9700

Offspring
60 Neal Street
London WC2H 9PA
Tel: 020 7497 2463

Prohibit
269 Elizabeth Street
New York, NY 10012
Tel: 212 219 1469

Size
33–34 Carnaby Street
London W1F 7DW
Tel: 020 7287 4016

Snaps
Sankt Pedersstaede 43
1453 Copenhagen K, Denmark
Tel: 45 33 32 39 11

Soletrader
72 Neal Street
London WC2H 9PA
Tel: 020 7836 6777

Sportie LA
7753 Melrose Avenue
Los Angeles, CA 90046
Tel: 323 651 1553

Ubiq
The Gallery
10th and Market Street
Philadelphia, PA 19110
Tel: 215 238 8005

Undefeated
112 1/2 La Brea Avenue
Los Angeles, CA 90036
Tel: 323 933 2251

INDEX (Figures in italics indicate captions)

CONTRIBUTORS

A vast majority of the shoes in this book are from a select group of collectors, most of whom are mentioned below. These shoes are extremely rare and valuable and we thank these people for letting us use them. A big thanks also goes to all who contributed their words, photographs, expertise and time to this project.

Charlie Ahearn wrote and directed the 1982 classic hip-hop movie *Wild Style*, which is now available on DVD. He recently collaborated with Jim Fricke of EMP to make *Yes, Yes, Y'all,* an oral history on the first decade of hip-hop, which includes photos by Ahearn shot before *Wild Style*. For more information, see www.wildstylethemovie.com.

John Connolly grew up and still lives in Liverpool. His infatuation with adidas began after purchasing adidas TRX in 1979 and he hasn't looked back since. John still trawls European cities for adidas,

but likens the advent of the internet (particularly ebay) to the 'Native American tribes being introduced to horses for hunting buffalo'.

Bobbito Garcia is probably the most famous trainer collector in the world. See www.sneakerfan.com/index2.htm for the inside scoop on this living legend.

Chris Hall is a famous ex-pro American Skate kid. He now spends his time searching for 'old skool' shoes as well as consulting for Nike, among others, on sneaker development.

Aaron Hawkins, store owner, product designer, photographer, and such, resides in Charlottesville, VA. As he best describes his own life story: Eeit gows a leetil sumfin' lyke deeess… yung buck, tryin' to buss a nut, grow'n up in tha V-A. Strayt gankin' owin da skatetilly, wrequ'n curbs-n-hoez frum hea 2 da villy, neva stowp fo no schule, no ruelz… jus'

pymp'n dem scrillaz aszif dae ain't no tomillaz. DEN, I browt a mess uh ideerrz up frum da souf, wif da lynz so pointa yo atteanshin-n-show't. I aiem dat maien da cawlid adawg da crusha. Numsain.

Fraser Moss is now best known for being co-founder of hip, young fashion brand 'You Must Create' (YMC). He cut his teeth, however, as one of the pioneers of 'old skool' trainer-sourcing back in the very early 1990s with his 'Professor Head' team of deadstock sourcers.

Marcus Ross spent his educational years in Bristol, sneaking into house parties where the likes of The Wild Bunch and DJ Kells were playing hip-hop and early house music. This introduction to 1980s music and style was followed by a sabbatical at art college. Having recently stepped down as fashion editor at *i-D* magazine after five years, he now works as a brand/trend consultant and freelance stylist.

Shaun Smith was also a contributor to the book *Sneakers: Size isn't Everything*, writing about the influence adidas has had on the English football Casual scene. There is nothing this man does not know about trainers. He also writes for the Everton Football Club fanzine, 'When Skies are Grey' and the magazines *Arena*, *Homme Plus* and *Sleaze Nation*.

Helen Sweeney-Dougan left her hometown of Glasgow at any early age in search of soul music and trainers. She has spent the last two decades travelling the world and during this time has worked as a consultant for many of the top brands as well her childhood heroes, Run DMC. A true trainer enthusiast and leading authority on subcultures, her home is now London where she spends her days talkin' shoes. Helen has set up her own trainer consultancy collective, which recruited many of the stars who have made this book what it is – they can be contacted at trainerfamily@hotmail.com

Johan Wirfält was Manmade on Earth™ in the late 1970s. These days he is a writer on music and street culture in the offices of the Swedish magazine *Bon*. At night he is most likely be found in various Stockholm DJ booths, making excuses for his mixes of the 1983 boogie disco he keeps referring to as 'funk', or at home with the love of his life, Jessica. The man would not call himself a sneaker collector, but he has been known to spend money on shoes he thinks are 'cool'. When asked about his favourite trainers, he'll mumble something about Delta Force 88s before conceding that 'At the end of the day, Chucks always did it for me'.

PICTURE CREDITS

The publishers would like to thank the following sources for their kind permission to reproduce the pictures in this book: pages 12/13 Jamal Shabazz excerpted from *Back in the Days* by Jamal Shabazz, Powerhouse Books; pages 16/18 David Corio; pages 20/21/22/23 Charlie Ahearn excerpted from *Yes Yes Y'all* DaCapo Press; page 24 Redferns; pages 26/31 Glen E. Friedman excerpted from *Fuck You Heroes*, Burning Flags Press; page78l Retna; page 78r Corbis; page 79l Rex; page 79r Kobal; page 80r Ronald Grant Archive; page 80r Kobal; page 81tl Godlis; page 81r Wireimage; page 81b Urban Image; page 84 Corbis; page 90 Empics; page 202 Timepix; page 288 Advertising Archives.

Thanks also to Vans, Vision, Dunlop, New Balance, P-F Flyers, Converse, Nike, adidas, Fila, Onitsuka, Puma, Reebok, DC Shoes, Tsubo, Pro-Keds and Diadora for their assistance with archive material.

ACKNOWLEDGEMENTS

Apologies for sounding like the Oscars, but it is truly important to thank those involved in such a big project as this. I would especially like to thank a few people without whom this book would not have been possible:

Firstly and foremost, thanks to Helen Sweeney-Dougan, who is featured in the book as a collector and who not only supplied her shoe collection for photography, but also helped considerably with her input, contacts, energy, commitment and dedication.

Big thanks to featured collectors Jeremy Howlett and Robert Brooks, who also allowed us to shoot their rare shoe collections. Thanks, too, to photographer David Gill (Gilly) who delivered above and beyond the call of duty with his artistic input, commitment and extreme work load.

Thanks to Shaun Smith and John Connolly for their excellent slant on the Casual culture in the U.K., which is shamefully under-covered by the press. Also for their valuable contacts in involving the legendary Mr Robert Wade Smith.

Thanks to Marcus 'the gent' Ross for his superb input in the fashion section, and to Charlie Ahearn, Aaron Hawkins and Glen E. Friedman for their input on the 'tribal culture' of our friends across the pond.

Thank you to the reknowned 'trainer heads' Robert Wade Smith and Bobbito, for sharing their trainer knowledge and stories with us.

Many thanks to those who I consider my good friends and who had a significant input – my Welsh compatriot Fraser 'Newport' Moss; my American, fellow 'trainer head', Chris Hall. Sincere thanks to Kevin 'South London' Hurry and Remi 'talks a lot' Kebaka, many of whose shoes we also see throughout the book.

Thanks to Johan Wirfält for his input and the contribution from his fellow Scandinavians Mikeadelica, Peter, Erik and Carmilla.

Love and thanks to Miss Tomo Robertson for her input and help. Cheers to Kerso for his help and time and the use of his 'mug-shot'. Also to Masahiro Minai, our Japanese collecting 'nut', the 'mad' DJ Cam, and Brian Whalen, for their time and effort.

Thanks to Chris Deeks for his Jabbar and other babies, Crusty for his 'monsters'. For their photographic input, cheers to David N. McIntyre for his RWS portrait and Mark McNulty for his shot of Graham Kerso Kerr.

Finally thanks to Carlton Publishing for commissioning the book in the first place and for having the dedication to keep the integrity of design. Many thanks also to: Jo Lee and Kirsty at Reebok, Robert at New Balance, Gina at Converse, Liz at Dunlop, Gavin at Pro-Keds, Charlie at Nike, Simon at Diadora and Rebecca at Asics. Cheers to Elena G, Zoë 'the wife', Lisa D and Penny at Carlton for all their help, time and patience. Special thanks to Judith at Carlton for loving her shoes and commissioning the book in the first place.

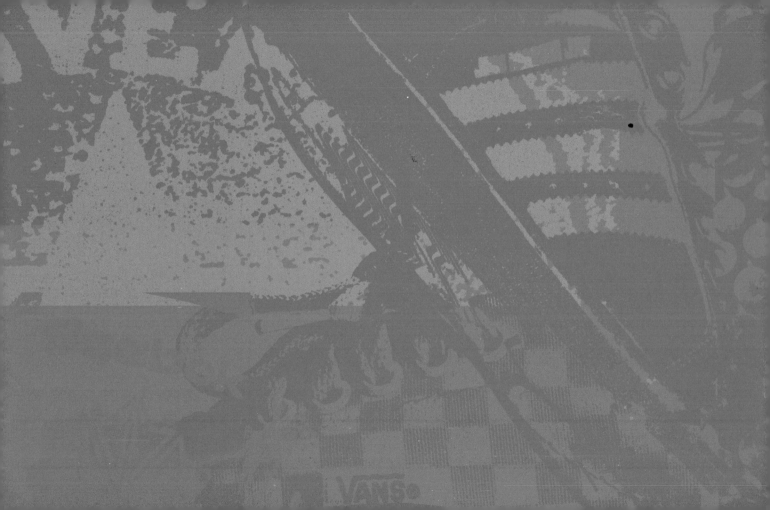